NEUROENDOCRINE TUMORS

A COMPREHENSIVE GUIDE TO DIAGNOSIS AND MANAGEMENT

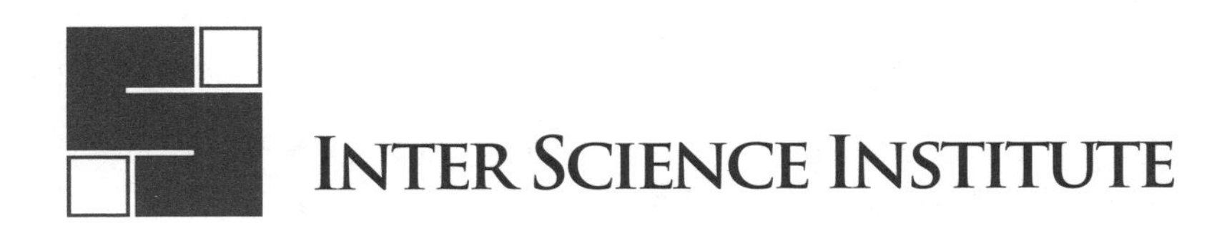

Aaron I. Vinik, MD, PhD
Thomas M. O'Dorisio, MD
Eugene A. Woltering, MD
Vay Liang W. Go, MD

Inter Science Institute GI Council

PREFACE

The GI Council of Inter Science Institute presents this comprehensive guide to diagnosis and management of neuroendocrine tumors to provide information and inspiration to all levels of clinicians, from novices to those professionally engaged in the field of neuroendocrine research, treatment, and analyses. This guidebook adds the new dimension of patient monitoring, not only through powerfully discriminating assays but through the recognition of clinical presentations and syndromes. This expertise is made possible by more than 150 years of cumulative experience of the advisory council.

Since the publication of the first GI Handbook in 1977 up to the current edition of *Neuroendocrine Tumors*, Inter Science Institute has been at the forefront of bridging the gap between academic medicine and the availability of the most current tests for patient diagnosis. In the intervening three and a half decades, unparalleled progress has been made both in the diagnosis and treatment of gastrointestinal, pancreatic, and neuroendocrine tumors.

This book is meant to be a *beacon* not only for listing tests but for all aspects of neuroendocrine tumors. Its publication represents a move from static text to the modern era of communication which allows for dynamic, continuously updating links to the ISI website, interscienceinstitute.com, as well as endotext.com as reference sources. Additionally, the book combines several references from the previous edition with an updated bibliography, in recognition of past contributions to the present.

Special thanks to our dedicated reviewers of this publication, Etta J. Vinik and Mia S. Tepper.

Finally, my appreciation and thanks to professors Vinik, Woltering, O'Dorisio, and Go for imparting their knowledge to the synergistic confluence that has given birth to this unique edition. Thank you, Arthur, Gene, O'Do, and Bill.

Gregg Mamikunian
Inter Science Institute 2006

Acknowledgments to the First Edition

The great majority of the gastrointestinal and pancreatic peptide hormones and polypeptide assays listed in this handbook would not have been even remotely possible had it not been for the tremendous generosity and cooperation of all the individuals listed below. Without their assistance, the establishment of the GI Hormones Laboratory at Inter Science Institute would not have been a reality.

Inter Science Institute gratefully acknowledges and thanks Professor V. Mutt of GI Hormones Laboratory of Karolinska Institute (Sweden) for his immense assistance and encouragement; Professor N. Yanaihara (Japan); Dr I.M. Samloff (USA); Professor J.C. Brown (Canada); Dr R. Geiger (Germany); Dr R.E. Chance (USA); Professor A.G.E. Pearse (England); Dr J.E. Hall (England); Dr R.I. Harvey (England) and Professor M. Bodanszky (USA).

Our sincerest appreciation to Professor John H. Walsh of the University of California at Los Angeles for his collaboration over the many years and his review and many suggestions regarding this presentation.

Finally, a special acknowledgment to Dr Herbert Gottfried of Inter Science Institute for his long and dedicated years in bringing the GI Hormones Laboratory into fruition.

Gregg Mamikunian
Inter Science Institute 1997
Reprinted from Inter Science Institute's *GI & Pancreatic Hormones and Polypeptides®* handbook, 1977.

Acknowledgments to the Second Edition

The current 1997 edition of the *GI, Pancreatic Hormones, Related Peptides and Compounds*® handbook presents comprehensive information for many rare procedures and tests that have been requested in the course of the past twenty-eight years.

The handbook reflects the tremendous advances that have been made since 1977. The number of tests offered has increased six-fold in addition to increasing specificity, sensitivity of antibodies, and purity of the standards. The protocols dealing with challenges and provocative testing has been expanded with the latest information. The section on the physiology of the GI and Pancreatic Hormones has been updated as an adjunct to the various procedures in the handbook.

Furthermore, the handbook covers a vast area of gastrointestinal, pancreatic, and other related procedures. Many of these procedures are clearly out of the realm of routine testing and request. On the other hand, quite a number of the procedures are indicators in the clinical confirmation of certain syndromes and disease states. Inter Science has witnessed the phenomenon over the years of the transformation of research-oriented procedures becoming useful, routine, and critical determining factors in the diagnosis and management of certain GI-related endocrinopathies.

A special acknowledgment to Alan C. Kacena for his dedication and service of twenty-five years at Inter Science Institute and in bringing the current edition of the GI Hormones handbook into reality.

Gregg Mamikunian
Inter Science Institute 1997
Reprinted from Inter Science Institute's *GI, Pancreatic Hormones, Related Peptides and Compounds*® handbook, 1997.

How to Use This Book

This book is designed for the medical practitioner; it is an educational tool as well as a practical manual for the diagnosis of patients with suspected neuroendocrine tumors and a variety of associated gastrointestinal disorders, guiding the physician to long-term follow-up. Conceptually, this text is more than a list of laboratory tests. It comprises two informational sections on gastroenteropancreatic tumors and clinical syndromes, both of which provide a step-by-step approach to possible diagnoses. Each diagnosis (with its CPT code provided) relates to appropriate tests in one of the three test sections: assays, profiles, and dynamic challenge tests. The assays are alphabetically arranged. Terminology and test names are cross-referenced in the comprehensive index.

Chapter 1

"Diagnosing and Treating Gastroenteropancreatic Tumors" describes the complexity of the problems involved with suspected neuroendocrine tumors. It then simplifies the problems by breaking them down under headings such as "Distinguishing Signs and Symptoms," "Diagnosis," "Biochemical Studies," and "Hormones and Peptides." Thus the physician is guided through a decision-making process from diagnosis to follow-up.

Chapter 2

"Clinical Syndromes" describes the signs, symptoms, and syndromes associated with excessive peptide amine release.

Chapter 3

"Assays" lists single tests alphabetically. The tests available from ISI are set out with clear and concise requirements. These include patient preparation, specimen collection, important precautions, shipping instructions, and CPT codes for insurance purposes.

Chapter 4

"Profiles" presents a collection of assays that should provide guidance to the diagnosing physician. Some of these tests are available locally, whereas others are available through ISI. This section also includes the requirements given in Chapter 4: patient preparation, specimen collection, important precautions, shipping instructions, and CPT codes for insurance purposes.

Chapter 5

"Dynamic Challenge Protocols" describes provocation tests. The drug doses outlined in these tests are recommendations only and should be reviewed and approved by the attending physician on a patient-by-patient basis. Dynamic challenge protocols can be dangerous and should be performed only under the direct and constant supervision of trained medical personnel who are familiar with expected and potentially unexpected responses to provocative testing.

Abbreviations are spelled out in the text the first time each is used. A list of abbreviations appears at the end of the book.

TABLE OF CONTENTS

Chapter 1

Chapter 2

TABLE OF CONTENTS

Chapter 3

Chapter 3 (cont.)

Chapter 4

TABLE OF CONTENTS

Chapter 4 (cont.)

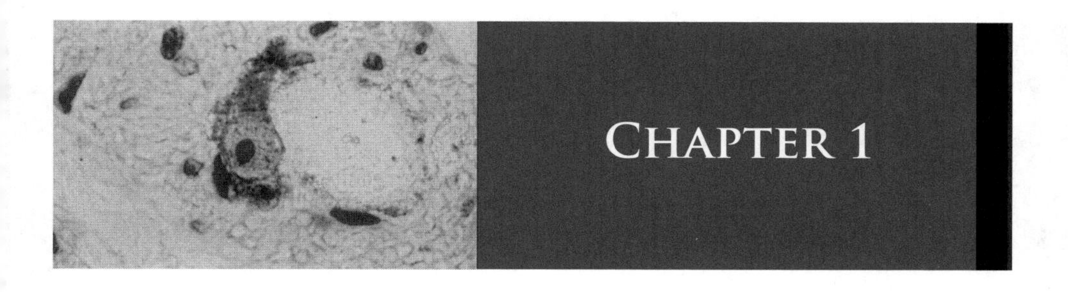

DIAGNOSING AND TREATING GASTROENTEROPANCREATIC TUMORS, INCLUDING ICD-9 CODES

GASTROENTEROPANCREATIC TUMORS

Endocrine tumors of the gastroenteropancreatic (GEP) axis (involving the gastrointestinal [GI] system, stomach, and pancreas) are comprised of cells capable of amine precursor uptake and decarboxylation, hence the prior name "APUDomas." The morphologic similarity of the APUD cells suggested a common embryologic origin, indicated by the term "protodifferentiated stem cell," now believed to derive from the endoderm and capable of giving rise to a variety of tumors **(Fig. 1-1)**.

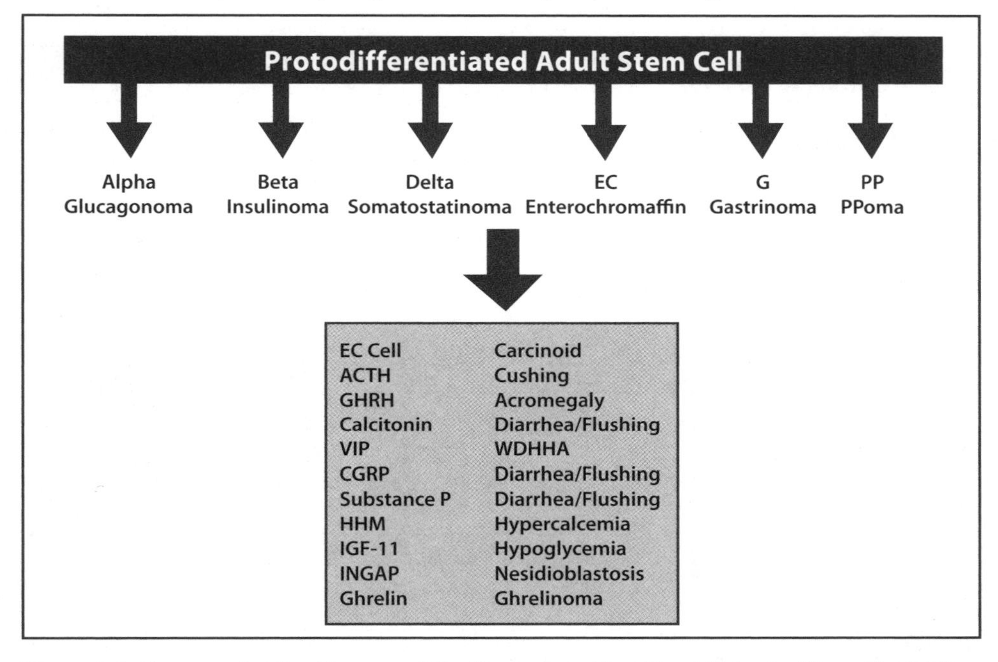

Figure 1-1. Neuroendocrine Tumors of the Gastrointestinal Tract (Adapted from Kvols LK, Perry RR, Vinik AI, et al. Neoplasms of the neuroendocrine system and neoplasms of the gastroenteropancreatic endocrine system. In: Bast RC Jr, Kufe DW, Pollock RE, et al, eds. Cancer Medicine, 6th ed. BC Dekker; 2003:1121-72.)

In some cases, multiple peptides or hormones are responsible for symptoms, and several organs and/or multiple tumors may be involved in the disease state, confounding the clinical diagnosis. To facilitate the diagnostic process, this text classifies GEP syndromes according to their secretory products and the clinical disorder they produce.

Carcinoid, gastrinoma, insulinoma, somatostatinoma, glucagonoma, and watery diarrhea (WDHHA) syndromes are described as individual syndromes according to their secretory hormones and peptides. Distinguishing signs and symptoms of each syndrome will further aid the diagnosis. These tumors can be subdivided into two main groups:

1. Orthoendocrine tumors secrete the normal product of the cell type (e.g., α-cell glucagon).
2. Paraendocrine tumors secrete a peptide or amine that is foreign to the organ or cell of origin.

Specific tumor syndromes, their clinical manifestations, and the tumor products are indicated in **(Table 1-1).**

Table 1-1. The Clinical Presentations, Syndromes, Tumor Types, Sites, and Hormones

Clinical Presentation	Syndrome	Tumor Type	Sites	Hormones
Flushing	Carcinoid	Carcinoid	Gastric, mid, and foregut, pancreas/ foregut, adrenal medulla	Serotonin, substance P, NKA, TCT, PP, CGRP, VIP
Diarrhea	Carcinoid	Carcinoid	As above	As above
	WDHHA	VIPoma	Pancreas, mast cells	VIP
	ZE	Gastrinoma	Pancreas, duodenum	Gastrin
	MCT	Medullary carcinoma	Thyroid, pancreas	Calcitonin
	PP	PPoma	Pancreas	PP
Diarrhea/Steatorrhea	Somatostatin	Somatostatinoma, neurofibromatosis	Pancreas, duodenum, bleeding GI tract	Somatostatin
Wheezing	Carcinoid	Carcinoid	Gut/pancreas, lung	Serotonin, substance P, chromogranin A
Dyspepsia, Ulcer Disease, Low pH on Endoscopy	ZE	Gastrinoma	Pancreas (85%), duodenum (15%)	Gastrin
Hypoglycemia	Whipple's triad	Insulinoma	Pancreas	Insulin
		Sarcomas	Retroperitoneal	IGF/binding protein
		Hepatoma	Liver	IGF
Dermatitis	Sweet's syndrome	Glucagonoma	Pancreas	Glucagon
	Pellagra	Carcinoid	Midgut	Serotonin
Dementia	Sweet's syndrome	Glucagonoma	Pancreas	Glucagon
Diabetes	Glucagonoma	Glucagonoma	Pancreas	Glucagon
	Somatostatin	Somatostatinoma	Pancreas	Somatostatin
Deep Venous Thrombosis	Somatostatin	Somatostatinoma	Pancreas	Somatostatin
Steatorrhea	Somatostatin	Somatostatinoma	Pancreas	Somatostatin
Cholelithiasis/ Neurofibromatosis	Somatostatin	Somatostatinoma	Pancreas	Somatostatin
Silent/Liver Metastases	PPoma	PPoma	Pancreas	PP
Acromegaly/ Gigantism	Acromegaly	Neuroendocrine tumors	Pancreas	GHRH
Cushing's	Cushing's	Neuroendocrine tumors	Pancreas	ACTH/CRF
Anorexia, Nausea, Vomiting	Hypercalcemia	Neuroendocrine tumors	Pancreas	PTHRP
Constipation, Abdominal Pain		VIPoma	Pancreas	VIP
Pigmentation		Neuroendocrine tumors	Pancreas	VIP
Postgastrectomy	Dumping, syncope, tachycardia, hypotension, borborygmus, explosive diarrhea, diaphoresis, mental confusion	None	Stomach/duodenum	Osmolarity, insulin, GLP

These are the common neuroendocrine tumors (NETs):

- Carcinoid
- Insulinoma
- PPoma
- Gastrinoma
- VIPoma
- Glucagonoma
- Somatostatinoma
- Ghrelinoma
- Multiple endocrine neoplasia types I and II (MEN-I and MEN-II)
- Other rare tumors

The great majority of these tumors are carcinoid tumors, accounting for more than half those presenting each year **(Fig. 1-2)**. The incidence of carcinoid has risen in the last 10 years, particularly those found in the stomach and ileum. Insulinomas, gastrinomas, and PPomas account for 17%, 15%, and 9%, respectively, whereas the rest remain around the 1% mark. These tumors are nicknamed "zebras" because of their rarity, but despite their infrequent occurrence, physicians are fascinated by their complexity and the unusual nature of their presentations. For the most part, endocrinologists make their living not by diagnosing and treating one of these tumors, but rather by *excluding* conditions that masquerade as NETs.

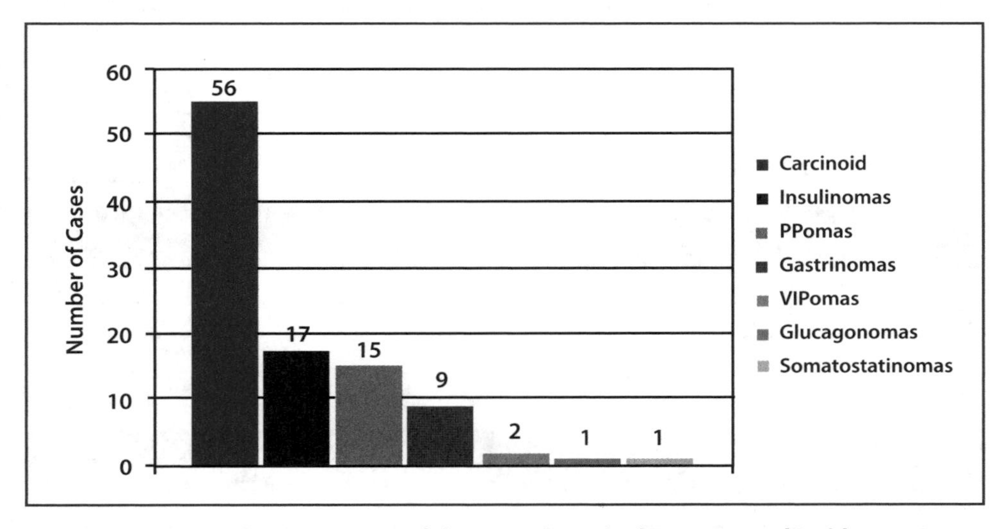

Figure 1-2. Neuroendocrine Tumors of the Gastrointestinal Tract: Annual Incidence 10 Cases per Million (From Vinik AI, Perry RR. Neoplasms of the gastroenteropancreatic endocrine system. In: Holland JF, Bast RC Jr, Morton DL, et al, eds. Cancer Medicine, vol. 1, 4th ed. Baltimore: Williams & Wilkins; 1997:1605-41.)

Characteristics of Neuroendocrine Tumors

- Rare
- Usually small (<1 cm)
- Slow growing (months to years, "cancer in slow motion")
- Usually metastasize to liver and bone before becoming symptomatic, often when tumor is larger than 2 cm
- Episodic expression; may be silent for years
- Often misdiagnosed; symptoms mimic commonplace conditions
- Complex diagnosis, rarely made clinically; requires sophisticated laboratory and scanning techniques

To facilitate the proper treatment regimen, diagnostic tests should be selected to
- Determine the peptide(s) or amines responsible for the symptoms
- Locate the site and cause of the abnormality
- Eliminate other possible causes and syndromes

ICD-9 CODE: Carcinoid Syndrome 259.2

ICD-9 CODES for Primary Carcinoid Tumor Sites

Foregut	Malignant	Benign	Uncertain Behavior	Unspecified
Duodenum	152.0	211.2	235.2	239.0
Lung	162.9	212.3	235.7	239.1
Stomach	151.9	211.1	235.2	239.0
Ovary	183.0	220	236.2	239.5
Thymus	164.0	212.6	235.8	239.8

Midgut	Malignant	Benign	Uncertain Behavior	Unspecified
Appendix	153.5	211.3	235.2	239.0
Colon	154.0	211.4	235.2	239.0
Ileum	152.0	211.2	235.2	239.0
Jejunum	152.1	211.2	235.2	239.0

Hindgut	Malignant	Benign	Uncertain Behavior	Unspecified
Rectum	154.1	211.4	235.2	239.0

ICD-9 CODES for Carcinoid Metastatic Sites

Lymph Nodes	Malignant
Supraclavicular	196.0
Abdominal	196.2
Mediastinal	196.1
Retroperitoneal	196.2

Carcinoid Organ	Metastatic Sites
Liver	197.7
Bone	198.5
Lung	162.0
Brain	191.9

(See Carcinoid Follow-Up Profile [Chapter 4] and Flushing Syndrome Tests [Chapter 4] for specific tests and CPT codes)

ICD-9 CODE: Glucagonoma

Malignant

Pancreas 157.9

Specified site–see Neoplasm by site, malignant

Unspecified site 157.4

Benign

Pancreas 211.6

Specified site–see Neoplasm by site, benign

Unspecified site 211.7

Uncertain behavior, neoplasm of the pancreas 235.5

ICD-9 CODE: Zollinger-Ellison Syndrome 251.5

ICD-9 CODE: Hepatoma

Malignant (M8170/3) 155.0

Benign (M8170/0) 211.5

Congenital (M8970/3) 155.0

Embryonal (M8970/3) 155.0

ICD-9 CODE: Whipple's Syndrome 040.2

ICD-9 CODE: Sweet's Syndrome 695.89

ICD-9 CODE: MEN-I and -II 258.0

ICD-9 CODE: Diarrhea 787.91

ICD-9 CODE: Functional Diarrhea 564.5

ICD-9 CODE: Achlorhydria 536.0

ICD-9 CODE: Gastrinoma (M8153/1)

ICD-9 CODES for Primary Sites

Sites	Malignant	Benign	Uncertain Behavior	Unspecified
Ampulla	156.2	211.5	235.3	239.0
Duodenum	152.0	211.2	235.2	239.0
Jejunum	152.1	211.2	235.2	239.0
Pancreas	157.9	211.6	235.5	239.0
Body	157.1	211.6	235.5	239.0
Head	157.0	211.6	235.5	239.0
Islet cell	157.4	211.7	235.5	239.0
Neck	157.8	211.6	235.5	239.0
Tail	157.2	211.6	235.5	239.0

ICD-9 CODES for Metastatic Sites

Sites	Malignant
Supraclavicular	196.0
Abdominal	196.2
Mediastinal	196.1
Retroperitoneal	196.2
Liver	197.7
Bone	198.5
Lung	162.0
Brain	191.9

(See GI–Neuroendocrine Tests [Chapter 4] for specific tests and CPT codes)

Carcinoid Tumors and the Carcinoid Syndrome

Carcinoid tumors are the most commonly occurring gut endocrine tumors. The prevalence of carcinoids is about 50,000 cases in any 1 year in the United States. The incidence is estimated to be approximately 1.5 cases per 100,000 of the general population (i.e., approximately 2500 new cases per year in the United States). Nonetheless, they account for 13% to 34% of all tumors of the small bowel and 17% to 46% of all malignant tumors of the small bowel. They derive from primitive stem cells known as Kulchitsky or enterochromaffin (EC) cells, originally described by Feyter as "wasser heller" or "clear water" cells and generally found in the gut wall.

Carcinoids may, however, occur in the bronchus, pancreas, rectum, ovary, lung, and elsewhere. The tumors grow slowly and often are clinically silent for many years before metastasizing. They frequently metastasize to the regional lymph nodes, liver, and, less commonly, to bone. The likelihood of metastases relates to tumor size. The incidence of metastases is less than 15% with a carcinoid tumor smaller than 1 cm but rises to 95% with tumors larger than 2 cm. In individual cases, size alone may not be the only determinant of lymphatic or distant spread. Lymphatic or vascular invasion, or spread into the fat surrounding the primary tumor, may be an indicator of a more aggressive tumor **(Table 1-2)**.

Table 1-2. Tumor Location and Frequency of Metastases (n=5468)

Gut	Location	Percentage of Tumors	Incidence of Metastases (%)
Foregut	Stomach	38	31
	Duodenum	21	33
	Lung	32.5	27
Midgut	Jejunum	2.3	70
	Ileum	17.6	70
	Appendix	7.6	35
	Colon	6.3	71
Hindgut		10	14

From Jensen RT. Carcinoid and pancreatic endocrine tumors: recent advances in molecular pathogenesis, localization, and treatment. Curr Opin Oncol. 12:368-77, 2000

The carcinoid syndrome occurs in less than 10% of patients with carcinoid tumors. It is especially common in tumors of the ileum and jejunum (i.e., midgut tumors) but also occurs with bronchial, ovarian, and other carcinoids. Tumors in the rectum (i.e., hindgut tumors) rarely occur in the carcinoid syndrome, even those that have widely metastasized. Tumors may be symptomatic only episodically, and their existence may go unrecognized for many years **(Fig. 1-3)**. The average time from onset of symptoms attributable to the tumor and diagnosis is just over 9 years, and diagnosis usually is made only after the carcinoid syndrome occurs. The distribution of carcinoids is Gaussian in nature. The peak incidence occurs in the sixth and seventh decades of life, but carcinoid tumors have also been reported in patients as young as 10 years of age and in those in their ninth decade.

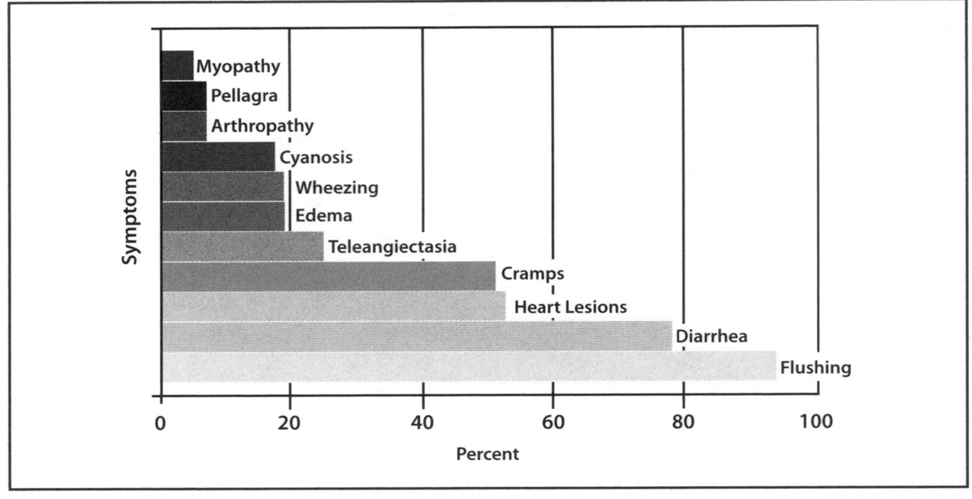

Figure 1-3. Frequency of Carcinoid Syndrome Symptoms

During the early stages, vague abdominal pain goes undiagnosed and invariably is ascribed to irritable bowel or spastic colon. At least one-third of patients with small bowel carcinoid tumors experience several years of intermittent abdominal pain before diagnosis. This pain can be due to obstruction (partial or intermittent) or to the development of intestinal angina, which in turn, may be due to bowel ischemia, especially in the postprandial period. Carcinoid tumors can present in a variety of ways. For example, duodenal tumors are known to produce gastrin and may present with the gastrinoma syndrome.

One of the more clinically useful classifications of carcinoid tumors is according to the classification of the primitive gut from which the tumor cells arise. These tumors derive from the stomach, foregut, midgut, and hindgut **(Table 1-3)**.

Table 1-3. Clinical and Biochemical Characteristics of Carcinoid Neuroendocrine Tumors

Tumor Location	Origin	Clinical Characteristics	Biochemical Characteristics
Gastric	Primary	Same as foregut	Same as foregut
	Secondary to achlorhydria	Pernicious anemia, atrophic gastritis, gastric polyps, gastrin <1000 pg/mL	
Foregut		Atypical carcinoid, ZE, acromegaly, Cushing's, etc.	5-HTP
Midgut		Classic carcinoid	Serotonin, substance P, CGRP, kinins, and peptides
Hindgut		Silent	Nonsecretory

Gastric Carcinoid

There are three types of gastric carcinoid tumors:

1. Type 1 gastric carcinoids are associated with achlorhydria, high gastrin levels, and multiple, small, relatively nonaggressive tumors. These tumors are more common in patients with achlorhydria accompanied by pernicious anemia and vitamin B_{12} deficiency, in which there is loss of gastric acid secretion causing impairment of the normal restraint mechanism suppressing gastrin production. Gastrin is trophic to EC cells in the stomach, and when levels rise above 1000 pg/mL, this constitutes a threshold for the induction of gastric carcinoid polyps and tumors.
2. Type 2 gastric carcinoids are associated with elevated gastric acid, high gastrin levels, and the Zollinger-Ellison (ZE) syndrome. These tumors are larger and have a higher propensity to metastasize than type 1 carcinoids of the stomach.
3. Type 3 gastric carcinoids are much larger than types 1 and 2 and have a high propensity to metastasize. These tumors are sporadic and may be associated with normal gastrin and gastric acid levels. This type of gastric carcinoid is most likely to cause tumor-related deaths.

The clinical picture of type 1 gastric carcinoid, most commonly identified in a patient with evidence of pernicious anemia, is characterized by the following:

- Premature graying of the hair
- Associated autoimmune disorders
- Antibodies to gastric parietal cells and intrinsic factor
- Achlorhydria or hypochlorhydria
- Neutral pH instead of the normal highly acidic pH
- Serum gastrin level greater than 1000 pg/mL

Foregut Carcinoid

Sporadic primary foregut tumors include carcinoids of the bronchus, stomach, first portion of the duodenum, pancreas, and ovaries. Midgut carcinoid tumors derive from the second portion of the duodenum, the jejunum, the ileum, and the right colon. Hindgut carcinoid tumors include those of the transverse colon, left colon, and rectum. This distinction assists in distinguishing a number of important biochemical and clinical differences among carcinoid tumors because the presentation, histochemistry, and secretory products are quite different (see Table 1-2). Foregut carcinoids are argentaffin negative. They have a low content of serotonin (5-hydroxytryptamine [5-HT]). They often secrete the serotonin precursor 5-hydroxytryptophan (5-HTP), histamine, and a multitude of polypeptide hormones. Their functional manifestations include carcinoid syndrome, gastrinoma syndrome, acromegaly, Cushing's disease, and a number of other endocrine disorders. Furthermore, they are unusual in that flushing tends to be of protracted duration, is often purplish or violet instead of the usual pink or red, and frequently results in telangiectasia and hypertrophy of the skin of the face and upper neck. The face may assume a leonine appearance after repeated episodes. It is not unusual for these tumors to metastasize to bone.

MIDGUT CARCINOID

Midgut carcinoids, in contrast, are argentaffin positive, have high serotonin content, rarely secrete 5-HTP, and often produce a number of other vasoactive compounds such as kinins, prostaglandins (PGs), and substance P. The clinical picture that results is the classic carcinoid syndrome of flushing and diarrhea with or without wheezing. These tumors may produce adrenocorticotropic hormone (ACTH) on rare occasions and infrequently metastasize to bone.

HINDGUT CARCINOID

Hindgut carcinoids are argentaffin negative, rarely contain serotonin, rarely secrete 5-HTP or other peptides, and usually are silent in their presentation. However, they may metastasize to bone. A further point of interest is that a gender variation is present when a carcinoid tumor coexists with MEN-I; more than two-thirds of the time the tumor is in the thymus in males, whereas in females, more than 75% of the time it is in the lung.

WHAT TO LOOK FOR

Distinguishing Signs and Symptoms

The major clinical manifestations of carcinoid tumors include the following:

- Cutaneous flushing (84%)
- GI hypermotility with diarrhea (70%)
- Heart disease (37%)
- Bronchial constriction/wheezing (17%)
- Myopathy (7%)
- Abnormal increase in skin pigmentation (5%)

Assessment of the concurrence of the two major symptoms of carcinoid tumors reveals that flushing and diarrhea occur simultaneously in 58% of cases, diarrhea without flushing in 15%, flushing without diarrhea in 5%, and neither flushing nor diarrhea as a symptom complex in 22%. The natural history of these tumors is illustrated in **Figure 1-4**. Invariably the patient has a long history of vague abdominal symptoms, a series of visits to his or her primary care practitioner, and referral to a gastroenterologist, often with a misdiagnosis of irritable bowel syndrome (IBS). These symptoms persist with a median latency to correct diagnosis of 9.2 years by which time the tumor has metastasized, causing flushing and diarrhea and progressing on its slow but relentless course until the patient dies. Clearly, a greater index of suspicion and a carcinoid tumor profile screen is warranted for all patients presenting with "traditional IBS symptoms." The diagnosis of metastases to the liver is generally more obvious but often still takes place only after a delay of many years. Even then, an incorrect diagnosis is not uncommon. Unless biopsy material is examined for the secretory peptide chromogranin, synaptophysin, or neuron-specific enolase (NSE), tumors may be labeled erroneously as adenocarcinoma, with a negative impact on physicians' attitudes regarding management and underestimation of prospects for survival.

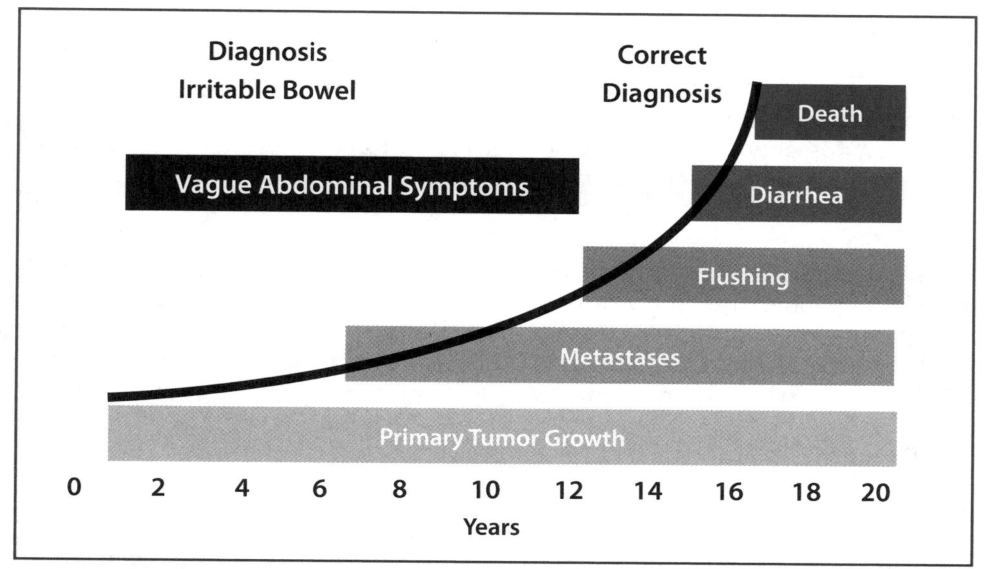

Figure 1-4. Natural History of Carcinoid Tumors (From Vinik A, Moattari AR. Use of somatostatin analog in management of carcinoid syndrome. Am J Dig Dis Sci. 34:14-27, 1989.)

Introduction to Chromogranins

Chromogranins belong to a unique family of secretory chromogranin and secretogranin proteins. Chromogranin A (CGA) is an acidic protein co-released with catecholamines during exocytosis from sympathetic nerve terminals and chromaffin cells.

Chromogranin A determination for diagnosis and follow-up in patients with gastroenteropancreatic endocrine tumors (GEP-ET) and MEN-I is considered the standard of care in many institutions. Although the absolute value of a single measurement of CGA is not a determinate of tumor bulk nor the presence or absence of metastasis, the trend in serial CGA levels over time has been proven to be a useful predictor of tumor growth. Changes in CGA levels of more than 25% over baseline are considered significant.

Serial measurements (every 3 to 6 months) of CGA levels in blood can be used to monitor the progression of a variety of gut-derived NETs. Serum CGA level is also an effective tumor marker in patients with pheochromocytoma. Increased levels strongly correlate with tumor mass. The concordance between CGA level and the results of iodine-131 meta-iodobenzylguanidine (^{131}I-MIBG) scintigraphy is high. A CGA level in the reference range is highly predictive of normal scintigraphy findings.

CGA levels may also be elevated in several other endocrine and nonendocrine diseases. It is well known that drugs that suppress gastric acid secretion can increase gastrin levels. Proton-pump inhibitors (PPI) are extensively used to treat patients with ZE syndrome, gastroesophageal reflux disease (GERD) or acid–peptic disease, but their long-term use can cause significant increases in gastrin levels and cause hypertrophy of the EC cells of the stomach. Enterochromaffin-like (ECL) cell hyperplasia secondary to hypergastrinemia also leads to increased levels of CGA in blood. Treatment with inhibitors of acid secretion, atrophic gastritis, and infection with *Helicobacter pylori* are common conditions leading to hypergastrinemia. These ECL cells are the precursor cells for the development of gastric carcinoids. An increase in CGA levels quickly follows the start of low dosages of PPI. Chronic high-dose PPI use can cause persistent elevations of CGA levels for months after discontinuing PPI therapy.

Renal insufficiency and severe hypertension have been associated with increases in CGA levels. Although antihypertensive drugs do not commonly interfere with the analysis of CGA levels, some false-positive results occur in the presence of renal impairment, hypergastrinemia, corticosteroid therapy, and the use of PPI. CGA has a circadian rhythm unrelated to plasma catecholamines; thus, collection of blood for serial measurement of CGA levels should be done at approximately the same time of day.

The Next Step

Diagnosis

The diagnosis of carcinoid tumors rests on a strong clinical suspicion in patients who present with flushing, diarrhea, wheezing, myopathy, and right-sided heart disease and includes appropriate biochemical confirmation and tumor localization studies.

Biochemical Studies

The rate-limiting step in carcinoid tumors for the synthesis of serotonin is the conversion of tryptophan into 5-HTP, catalyzed by the enzyme tryptophan hydroxylase. In midgut tumors, 5-HTP is rapidly converted to serotonin by the enzyme aromatic amino acid decarboxylase (dopa-decarboxylase). Serotonin is either stored in the neurosecretory granules or may be secreted directly into the vascular compartment. Most of the secreted serotonin is taken up by platelets and stored in their secretory granules. The rest remains free in the plasma, and circulating serotonin is then largely converted into the urinary metabolite 5-hydroxyindoleacetic acid (5-HIAA) by the enzymes monoamine oxidase and aldehyde dehydrogenase. These enzymes are abundant in the kidney, and the urine typically contains large amounts of 5-HIAA.

In patients with foregut tumors, the urine contains relatively little 5-HIAA but large amounts of 5-HTP. It is presumed that these tumors are deficient in dopa-decarboxylase; this deficiency impairs the conversion of 5-HTP into serotonin, leading to 5-HTP secretions into the vascular compartment. Some 5-HTP, however, is converted to serotonin and 5-HIAA, producing modest increases in levels of these metabolites. The normal range for 5-HIAA secretion is 2 to 8 mg per 24 hours, and the quantitation of serotonin and all of its metabolites usually permits the detection of 84% of patients with carcinoid tumors. No single measurement detects all cases of carcinoid syndrome, although the urine 5-HIAA appears to be the best screening procedure. Other peptides involved include substance P, neuropeptide K, pancreatic polypeptide (PP), and CGA.

Neuroendocrine tumors are characterized by their capacity to synthesize, store, and release hormonal products. These substances are stored in neurosecretory vesicles together with CGA. The concentration of CGA in plasma is thought to reflect the neuroendocrine differentiation of the tumor and the total tumor burden as well as to be useful as a means of measuring response to treatment. The "value" of CGA for diagnosis and follow-up of NETs has a sensitivity of 62.9% with specificity of 98.4%; levels are higher in secreting versus nonsecreting tumors (7% vs 45%) and are related to the extent of metastases. In nonsecreting tumors, the positive predictive value for the presence of metastases is 100%, but the negative predictive value is only 50%. In MEN-I, a high value predicts the presence of a pancreatic tumor with 100% specificity, but the sensitivity is only 59%. During follow-up, the concordance of tumor growth and CGA is 80%, better than that with serotonin (81% vs 54%). Thus, owing to its high specificity, CGA determination may help to discriminate the endocrine character of an NET and to establish a pancreatic tumor in MEN-I syndrome. Serial measurements are also useful for evaluating response to treatment.

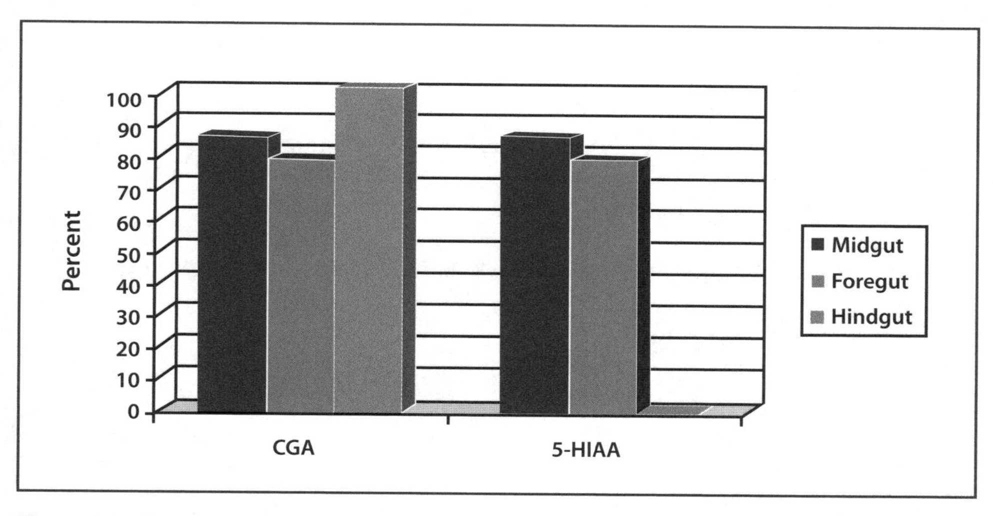

Figure 1-5. Chromogranin A Versus 5-HIAA in Neuroendocrine Tumors (From Vinik AI. Carcinoid tumors. In: DeGroot LJ, Jameson JL, eds. Endocrinology, vol. 3, 4th ed. Philadelphia, PA: WB Saunders; 2001:2533-58.)

Figure 1-5 shows the percent positivity of CGA versus 5-HIAA in the different carcinoids. CGA is positive 80% to 100% of the time in fore-, mid-, and hindgut tumors, whereas 5-HIAA detects a little more than 70% of midgut tumors, reveals only 30% of foregut tumors, and fails to recognize the presence of a hindgut carcinoid tumor. Evaluating PP levels in conjunction with CGA levels may further enhance this sensitivity. Both markers were measured in 68 patients (28 functioning and 40 nonfunctioning tumors). CGA sensitivity was 96% in functioning tumors and 75% in nonfunctioning tumors, and 74% in pancreatic and 91% in gastrointestinal tumors. Specificity was 89%.

In contrast to CGA alone, PP sensitivity for NETs was approximately 50%, but combining the two markers increased sensitivity for all tumors to greater than 95%. More specifically, the gain in detection of pancreatic tumors was 93% with CGA and PP versus 68% using CGA alone. It seems reasonable to recommend using both markers under these circumstances. There are, however, always caveats. Gastric parietal cell antibodies neutralize acid secretion thereby unbridling the G cell to produce gastrin that is trophic to the gastric ECL cells. Following a period of progressive hypertrophy, these ECL cells can transform into gastric carcinoid. Measurement of gastrin and CGA, but not NSE and 5-HIAA, is a means of evaluating the ECL mass. This is particularly useful in therapeutic decision-making with regard to doing an antrectomy or simply following conservatively and removing carcinoid polyps as they arise. Of course, this raises the issue of whether reported elevations in CGA in people taking PPI are truly false-positive or reflect ECL hyperplasia. Nonetheless, all evidence points to the combined measurement of the following markers:

- CGA
- PP
- Gastrin
- Gastric pH

These measurements are a very effective means of discovering a NET, identifying its probable site of origin, and monitoring response to intervention. In carcinoid tumors, neurotensin is elevated in 43% of patients, substance P in 32%, motilin in 14%, somatostatin in 5%, and vasoactive intestinal peptide (VIP) rarely.

Common amines and peptides produced by carcinoids that cause symptoms are as follows:

- Serotonin
- Histamine
- Substance P

The following constitute the best clinical practice panel of markers for diagnosis and follow-up of carcinoid tumors:

- CGA
- 5-HIAA
- Gastrin
- Serotonin
- Pancreastatin
- Neurokinin A (NKA; substance K)

In patients who are not responding to octreotide clinically or biochemically or in those who exhibit tumor progression, measurement of the octreotide level will help determine appropriateness of drug dosing. Quantification of plasma hormonal responses to octreotide suppression may help in the prediction of long-term responses to therapy.

ICD-9 CODE: Carcinoid Syndrome 259.2

ICD-9 CODES for Carcinoid Primary Tumor Sites

Foregut	Malignant	Benign	Uncertain Behavior	Unspecified
Duodenum	152.0	211.2	235.2	239.0
Lung	162.9	212.3	235.7	239.1
Stomach	151.9	211.1	235.2	239.0
Ovary	183.0	220.0	236.2	239.5
Thymus	164.0	212.6	235.8	239.8

Midgut	Malignant	Benign	Uncertain Behavior	Unspecified
Appendix	153.5	211.3	235.2	239.0
Colon	154.0	211.4	235.2	239.0
Ileum	152.0	211.2	235.2	239.0
Jejunum	152.1	211.2	235.2	239.0

Midgut	Malignant	Benign	Uncertain Behavior	Unspecified
Rectum	154.1	211.4	235.2	239.0

ICD-9 CODES for Carcinoid Metastatic Sites

Lymph Nodes	Malignant
Supraclavicular	196.0
Abdominal	196.2
Mediastinal	196.1
Retroperitoneal	196.2

Carcinoid Organ	Metastastatic Sites
Liver	197.7
Bone	198.5
Lung	162.0
Brain	191.9

(See Carcinoid Follow-Up Profile [Chapter 4] and Flushing Syndrome Tests [Chapter 4] for specific tests and CPT codes)

Insulinomas

The classic description of insulinoma is of Whipple's triad, which includes symptoms of hypoglycemia with a low blood glucose concentration relieved by the ingestion of glucose. These tumors are most commonly benign (90%) and can be located anywhere within the pancreas. Insulinomas are associated with a memory rule known as "the rule of tens," which refers to the following characteristics: 10% are malignant; 10% are ectopic; and 10% are related to the MEN-I syndrome. Removal of the tumor, which is invariably in the pancreas, is curative in more than 90% of cases.

Adult-onset nesidioblastosis is a rare condition in which islets become hypertrophied and produce excess insulin. The diagnostic differentiation of an insulinoma from adult-onset nesidioblastosis is possible only by histologic evaluation of sufficient pancreatic tissue; fine needle biopsy does not obtain a specimen of adequate quantity. In the newborn, hypoglycemia and excess insulin production can be caused by nesidioblastosis; insulinomas are rare in this age group.

What to Look For

Distinguishing Signs and Symptoms

The major symptoms of an insulinomas are those of hypoglycemia, which can be adrenergic:

- Nervousness
- Sweating
- Palpitations
- Diaphoresis (profuse sweating)
- Circumoral tingling

Central nervous system symptoms include the following:

- Blurred vision
- Confusion
- Disorientation
- Memory loss leading to coma
- Stupor
- If chronic, dementia

The Next Step

The blood glucose level alone is not diagnostic for insulinoma, nor in general is the absolute insulin level elevated in all cases of organic hyperinsulinism (see Hypoglycemia in Chapter 2). The standard diagnostic test remains a 72-hour fast while the patient is closely observed. More than 95% of cases can be diagnosed based on their response to this test. Serial glucose and insulin levels are obtained every 4 hours over the 72-hour period until the patient becomes symptomatic. When symptoms occur, obtain insulin, glucose, and C-peptide levels. Because the absolute insulin level is not elevated in all patients with insulinomas, a normal level does not rule out the disease; however, a fasting insulin level of greater than 24 μU/mL is found in approximately 50% of patients with insulinoma. This is strong evidence in favor of the diagnosis. Values of insulin greater than 7 μU/mL after a more prolonged fast in the presence of a blood glucose level less than 40 mg/dL are also highly suggestive. A refinement in the interpretation of glucose and insulin levels has been established by determining the ratio of insulin levels in microunits per milliliter to the concomitant glucose level in milligrams per deciliter. An insulin/glucose ratio greater than 0.3 has been found in virtually all patients proven to have an insulinoma or other islet cell disease causing organic hyperinsulinism. Calculating the amended insulin/glucose ratio as follows can increase the accuracy of the test:

amended ratio = insulin (μU/mL)/glucose (mg/dL) – 30 normal <50

If the amended ratio is greater than 50, then organic hyperinsulinism is certain. Measurements of proinsulin and C-peptide have proven to be valuable in patients suspected of having organic hypoglycemia. Normally, the circulating proinsulin concentration accounts for less than 22% of the insulin immunoreactivity but is greater than 24% in more than 90% of individuals with insulinomas. Furthermore, a proinsulin level greater than 40% is highly suspicious for a malignant islet cell tumor. The C-peptide level is useful in ruling out fictitious hypoglycemia from self-administration of insulin. Commercial insulin preparations contain no C-peptide, and combined with high insulin levels, low C-peptide levels confirm the diagnosis of self-administration of insulin. High-performance liquid chromatography to characterize the insulin species found in the blood was useful before the advent of recombinant human insulin, which is not distinguishable from native insulin. Patients who take sulfonylureas surreptitiously may have increased insulin and C-peptide values soon after ingestion, but chronic use will result in hypoglycemia without increased insulin or C-peptide levels. Only an index of suspicion and measurement of urine sulfonylureas will lead to the correct diagnosis. A variety of insulin stimulation and suppression tests were used before precise and accurate insulin measurements were available. Each had its limitations, and all are currently considered obsolete. The insulin response to secretin stimulation (2 U/kg intravenously; peak response in 1–5 minutes) is a valuable measure to differentiate multiple adenomas from nesidioblastosis and single adenomas. The normal maximal increase is 74 μU/mL, whereas in single adenomas it is only 17 μU/mL, in nesidioblastosis it is 10 μU/mL, and in two patients with multiple B-cell adenomas and hyperplasia, the increases were 214 and 497 μU/mL. Patients with single adenomas and nesidioblastosis do not respond to secretin, whereas those with multiple adenomas or hyperplasia have an excessive insulin response to the administration of secretin.

Hormones and Peptides

- Insulin
- Proinsulin
- C-peptide

The standard diagnostic test is a 72-hour fast while the patient is closely observed. More than 95% of cases can be diagnosed based on responses to a 72-hour fast (see 72-Hour Supervised Fast for the Diagnosis of Insulinoma, Chapter 5). Symptomatic hypoglycemia must be accompanied by a correspondingly low blood glucose value (<50 mg/dL) with relief of symptoms by the administration of glucose.

ICD-9 CODE: Insulinomas M8151/0

- Malignant (M8151/3)
  - Pancreas 157.4
  - Unspecified site 157.4
  - Specified site–see Neoplasm by site, malignant
- Benign, unspecified site 211.7
- Uncertain behavior, neoplasm of pancreas 235.5

ICD-9 CODES for Primary Islet Cell Sites

Sites	Malignant	Benign	Uncertain Behavior	Unspecified
Ampulla	156.2	211.5	235.3	239.0
Duodenum	152.0	211.2	235.2	239.0
Jejunum	152.1	211.2	235.2	239.0
Pancreas	157.9	211.6	235.5	239.0
Body	157.1	211.6	235.5	239.0
Head	157.0	211.6	235.5	239.0
Islet cell	157.4	211.7	235.5	239.0
Neck	157.8	211.6	235.5	239.0
Tail	157.2	211.6	235.5	239.0

ICD-9 CODES for Metastatic Sites

Sites	Malignant
Supraclavicular	196.0
Abdominal	196.2
Mediastinal	196.1
Retroperitoneal	196.2
Liver	197.7
Bone	198.5
Lung	162.0
Brain	191.9

(See 72-Hour Supervised Fast for the Diagnosis of Insulinoma [Chapter 5], Oral Glucose Tolerance Test for Diabetes, Insulinoma, Impaired Glucose Tolerance, Metabolic Syndrome, PCOS, Reactive Hypoglycemia, and Acromegaly [Chapter 5], Diabetes Type 1 Screen [Chapter 4], and Hypoglycemia/Insulinoma Screening Test [Chapter 4] for specific tests and CPT codes)

Glucagonoma Syndrome

In 1966, McGavran and colleagues called attention to a syndrome that included acquired diabetes and glucagon-producing tumors. Because these tumors usually were accompanied by a very characteristic skin rash, the syndrome is also known as the 4D syndrome, which stands for dermatosis, diarrhea, deep venous thrombosis (DVT), and depression.

What to Look For

Distinguishing Signs and Symptoms

- Characteristic rash (necrolytic migratory erythema [NME]) (82%)
- Painful glossitis
- Angular stomatitis
- Normochromic normocytic anemia (61%)
- Weight loss (90%)
- Mild diabetes mellitus (80%)
- Hypoaminoacidemia
- DVT (50%)
- Depression (50%)

In a study of 1366 consecutive adult autopsies, a tumor frequency of 0.8% was found. All tumors were adenomas, and all contained histochemically defined glucagon cells. None of the tumors had been suspected during life. Although these adenomas contained glucagon, it is not known whether they were overproducing or even secreting glucagon. The incidence in vivo is probably 1% of all NETs.

Features of the Necrolytic Migratory Erythematous Rash

The NME rash of the glucagonoma syndrome has a characteristic distribution. It usually is widespread, but major sites of involvement are the perioral and perigenital regions along with the fingers, legs, and feet. It may also occur in areas of cutaneous trauma. The basic process in the skin seems to be one of superficial epidermal necrosis, fragile blister formation, crusting, and healing with hyperpigmentation. Skin biopsy specimens usually show small bullae containing acantholytic epidermal cells as well as neutrophils and lymphocytes. The adjacent epidermis usually is intact, and the dermis contains a lymphocytic perivascular infiltrate. Different stages of the cutaneous lesions may be present simultaneously. Biopsy examination of a fresh skin lesion may be the most valuable aid in suggesting the diagnosis of glucagonoma syndrome, but repeated biopsy samples may be necessary to confirm the diagnosis. A painful glossitis manifested by an erythematous, mildly atrophic tongue has been associated with the cutaneous lesions.

Two other features of the syndrome are noteworthy:

1. A high rate of thromboembolic complications, particularly pulmonary embolism and the unexplained occurrence of arterial thrombosis. Unexplained thromboembolic disease should alert one to the possibility of glucagonoma. (In some studies, anticoagulation therapy with warfarin has been ineffective). Most

authors recommend heparin-based therapy for patients with this complication of glucagonoma.
2. Depression and other psychiatric disturbances.

Other metabolic disorders associated with cutaneous lesions may closely resemble the NME of the glucagonoma syndrome. These include:

- Acrodermatitis enteropathica
- Zinc deficiency induced by hyperalimentation
- Essential fatty acid deficiency
- Dermatosis of protein calorie malnutrition of kwashiorkor
- Pellagra resulting from niacin deficiency

Cutaneous manifestations associated with malabsorptive states often are nonspecific, affecting approximately 20% of patients with steatorrhea.

Glucose Intolerance

Glucose intolerance in the glucagonoma syndrome may relate to tumor size. Fasting plasma glucagon levels tend to be higher in patients with large hepatic metastases than in those without hepatic metastases, and all patients with large hepatic metastases have glucose intolerance. Massive hepatic metastases may decrease the ability of the liver to metabolize splanchnic glucagon, thus increasing peripheral plasma glucagon levels. Glucagon may not directly induce hyperglycemia, however, unless metabolism of glucose by the liver is directly compromised.

The Next Step

Measure plasma glucagon concentrations by radioimmunoassay. In patients with glucagonomas, fasting plasma glucagon concentrations may be as high as 2100 ± 334 pg/mL. These levels are markedly higher than those reported in normal, fasting subjects (i.e., <150 pg/mL) or in those with other disorders causing hyperglucagonemia, including diabetes mellitus, burn injury, acute trauma, bacteremia, cirrhosis, renal failure, or Cushing's syndrome, in which fasting plasma glucagon concentrations often are elevated but remain less than 500 pg/mL.

Hormones and Peptides

As with other islet cell neoplasms, glucagonomas may overproduce multiple hormones:

- Glucagon
- Insulin
- CGA
- PP
- Parathyroid hormone (PTH)
- Substances with PTH-like activity
- Gastrin
- Serotonin
- VIP and melanocyte-stimulating hormone (MSH), in that order of frequency

Measure the following:

- Plasma glucagon
- Insulin

- ACTH, PP
- Gastrin
- Serotonin
- VIP
- PTH
- Parathyroid hormone–related peptide (PTHRP)

ICD-9 CODE: Glucagonoma

Malignant
- Pancreas 157.4
- Unspecified site 157.4
- Specified site–see Neoplasm by site, malignant

Benign
- Pancreas 211.7
- Unspecified site 211.7

Uncertain behavior, neoplasm of the pancreas 235.5

ICD-9 CODES for Primary Islet Cell Tumor Sites

Sites	Malignant	Benign	Uncertain Behavior	Unspecified
Ampulla	156.2	211.5	235.3	239.0
Duodenum	152.0	211.2	235.2	239.0
Jejunum	152.1	211.2	235.2	239.0
Pancreas	157.9	211.6	235.5	239.0
Body	157.1	211.6	235.5	239.0
Head	157.0	211.6	235.5	239.0
Islet cell	157.4	211.7	235.5	239.0
Neck	157.8	211.6	235.5	239.0
Tail	157.2	211.6	235.5	239.0

ICD-9 CODES for Islet Cell Tumor Metastatic Sites

Sites	Malignant
Supraclavicular	196.0
Abdominal	196.2
Mediastinal	196.1
Retroperitoneal	196.2
Liver	197.7
Bone	198.5
Lung	162.0
Brain	191.9

(See Glucagon [Chapter 3] and GI–Neuroendocrine Tests (Chapter 4) for specific tests and CPT codes)

Reference

1. McGavran MH, Unger RH, Recant L, et al. A glucagon-secreting α-cell carcinoma of the pancreas. N Engl J Med. June 23;274(25):1408-13, 1966.

SOMATOSTATINOMA

Somatostatin (somatotropin release–inhibiting factor [SRIF]) is a tetradecapeptide that inhibits numerous endocrine and exocrine secretory functions. Almost all gut hormones that have been studied are inhibited by SRIF, including insulin, PP, glucagon, gastrin, secretin, gastric inhibitory polypeptide (GIP), and motilin. In addition to inhibition of the endocrine secretions, SRIF has direct effects on a number of target organs. For example, it is a potent inhibitor of basal and PG-stimulated gastric acid secretion. It also has marked effects on GI transit time, intestinal motility, and absorption of nutrients from the small intestine. The major effect in the small intestine appears to be a delay in the absorption of fat and reduced absorption of calcium.

WHAT TO LOOK FOR

Distinguishing Signs and Symptoms

The salient features of the somatostatinoma syndrome are as follows:

- Diabetes
- Diarrhea/steatorrhea
- Gallbladder disease (cholelithiasis and dysmotility)
- Hypochlorhydria
- Weight loss

Diagnostic Markers

Plasma Somatostatin-Like Immunoreactivity

The mean somatostatin-like immunoreactivity (SLI) concentration in patients with pancreatic somatostatinoma was 50 times higher than normal (range, 1–250 times). Intestinal somatostatinomas, however, present differently and have only slightly elevated or normal SLI concentrations **(Table 1-4).**

Table 1-4. Comparison of Pancreatic and Intestinal Somatostatinoma

Pancreatic Somatostatinoma	Intestinal Somatostatinoma
SLI 50x higher than normal (range, 1–250 times)	SLI slightly elevated or normal
75% of patients have diabetes	11% of patients have diabetes
Tumors are large and destroy part of pancreas	Tumors are relatively small
59% of patients have gallbladder disease	27% of patients have gallbladder disease
Diarrhea and steatorrhea are common	Diarrhea and steatorrhea are rare
Weight loss in one third of patients	Weight loss in one fifth of patients
Acid secretion inhibited in 87% of patients	Acid secretion inhibited in 12% of patients
	Café-au-lait spots
	Neurofibromatosis
	Paroxysmal hypertension

The Next Step

Diabetes Mellitus

When pancreatic and intestinal tumors result in diabetes, the diabetes is relatively mild and can usually be controlled by diet with or without oral hypoglycemic agents or by small doses of insulin. It is not clear, however, whether the differential inhibition of insulin and diabetogenic hormones can explain the usually mild degree of diabetes and the rarity of ketoacidosis in patients with somatostatinoma. Replacement of functional islet cell tissue by pancreatic tumor may be another reason for the development of diabetes in most patients with pancreatic somatostatinoma, contrasting with the low incidence of diabetes in patients with intestinal tumors. Pancreatic tumors are usually large and therefore destroy substantial portions of the organ.

Gallbladder Disease

The high incidence of gallbladder disease in patients with somatostatinoma and the absence of such an association in any other islet cell tumor suggest a causal relation between gallbladder disease and somatostatinoma. Infusion of somatostatin into normal human subjects has been shown to inhibit gallbladder emptying, suggesting that somatostatin-mediated inhibition of gallbladder emptying (dysmotility) may cause the observed high rate of gallbladder disease in patients with somatostatinoma. This theory is supported by the observation of massively dilated gallbladders without stones or other pathology in patients with somatostatin-secreting tumors.

Diarrhea and Steatorrhea

Diarrhea consisting of 3 to 10 frequently foul-smelling stools per day and/or steatorrhea of 20 to 76 g of fat per 24 hours is common in patients with pancreatic somatostatinoma, even with a controlled amount of fat in the diet. This could result from the effects of high levels of somatostatin within the pancreas serving as a paracrine mediator to inhibit exocrine secretion or, alternatively, from duct obstruction caused by the somatostatinoma. In some cases, the severity of diarrhea and steatorrhea parallels the course of the disease, worsening as the tumor advances and metastatic disease spreads and improving after tumor resection. Somatostatin has been shown to inhibit the pancreatic secretion of proteolytic enzymes, water, bicarbonate, and gallbladder motility. In addition, it inhibits the absorption of lipids. All but 1 patient with diarrhea and steatorrhea have had high plasma somatostatin concentrations. The rarity of diarrhea and/or steatorrhea in patients with intestinal somatostatinomas may result from the lower SLI levels seen in patients with that condition.

Hypochlorhydria

Infusion of somatostatin has been shown to inhibit gastric acid secretion in human subjects. Thus, hypochlorhydria in patients with somatostatinoma, in the absence of gastric mucosal abnormalities, is likely to result from elevated somatostatin concentrations. Basal and stimulated acid secretion was inhibited in 87% of patients with pancreatic tumors tested but in only 12% of patients with intestinal tumors.

Weight Loss

Weight loss ranging from 9 to 21 kg over several months occurred in one third of patients with pancreatic tumors and one fifth of patients with intestinal tumors. The weight loss may relate to malabsorption and diarrhea, but in small intestinal tumors, anorexia, abdominal pain, and yet unexplained reasons may be relevant.

Associated Endocrine Disorders

Approximately 50% of all patients have other endocrinopathies in addition to their somatostatinoma. Occurrence of MEN-I has been recognized in patients with islet cell tumors, and MEN-II or MEN-III syndromes are present in association with pheochromocytomas and neurofibromatosis, respectively. It seems that an additional dimension of the duct-associated tumors is MEN-II. Secretion of different hormones by the same islet cell tumor, sometimes resulting in two distinct clinical disorders, is now being recognized with increasing frequency. These possibilities should be considered during endocrine workups of patients with islet cell tumors and their relatives.

Tumor Location

Of the reported primary tumors, 60% were found in the pancreas and 40% in the duodenum or jejunum. Of the pancreatic tumors, 50% were located in the head, and 25% in the tail, and the remaining tumors either infiltrated the whole pancreas or were found in the body. Regarding extrapancreatic locations, approximately 50% originate in the duodenum, approximately 50% originate in the ampulla, and rarely one is found in the jejunum. Thus, approximately 60% of somatostatinomas originate in the upper intestinal tract, probably a consequence of the relatively large number of delta (somatostatin) cells in this region.

Tumor Size

Somatostatinomas tend to be large, similar to glucagonomas but unlike insulinomas and gastrinomas, which, as a rule, are small. Within the intestine, tumors tend to be smaller than somatostatinomas located elsewhere. Symptoms associated with somatostatinomas and glucagonomas are less pronounced and probably do not develop until very high blood levels of the respective hormones have been attained. As a result, somatostatinomas and glucagonomas are likely to be diagnosed late in the course of the disease.

Incidence of Malignancy

Eighty percent (80%) of patients with pancreatic somatostatinomas had metastases at diagnosis, and 50% with intestinal tumors had evidence of metastatic disease. Metastasis to the liver is most frequent, and regional lymph node involvement and metastases to bone are less so. Thus, in approximately 70% of cases, metastatic disease is present at diagnosis. This is similar to the high incidence of malignancy in glucagonoma and in gastrinoma, but it is distinctly different from the low incidence of malignant insulinoma. The high prevalence of metastatic disease in somatostatinoma also may be a consequence of late diagnosis but apparently is not dependent on the tissue of origin.

Somatostatin-Containing Tumors Outside the GI Tract

Somatostatin has been found in many tissues outside the GI tract. Prominent among those are the hypothalamic and extrahypothalamic regions of the brain, the peripheral nervous system (including the sympathetic adrenergic ganglia), and the C cells of the thyroid gland. Not surprisingly, therefore, high concentrations of somatostatin have been found in tumors originating from these tissues. Some patients exhibited the clinical somatostatinoma syndrome.

Elevated plasma SLI concentrations also have been reported in patients with small cell lung cancer. In one patient with metastatic bronchial oat cell carcinoma, the tumor caused Cushing's syndrome, diabetes, diarrhea, steatorrhea, anemia, and weight loss, and the patient had a plasma SLI concentration 20 times greater than normal. A patient with a bronchogenic carcinoma presenting with diabetic ketoacidosis and high levels of SLI (>5000 pg/mL) has been reported. Pheochromocytomas and catecholamine-producing extra-adrenal paragangliomas are other examples of endocrine tumors that produce and secrete somatostatin in addition to other hormonally active substances. One fourth of 37 patients with pheochromocytomas had elevated SLI levels.

Tumors are identified as somatostatinomas by the demonstration of elevated tissue concentrations of SLI and/or prevalence of D cells by immunocytochemistry or demonstration of elevated plasma SLI concentrations. Thus, events leading to the diagnosis of somatostatinoma usually occur in reverse order. In other islet cell tumors, the clinical symptoms and signs usually suggest the diagnosis, which then is established by demonstration of diagnostically elevated blood hormone levels, following which efforts are undertaken to localize the tumors.

The diagnosis of somatostatinoma at a time when blood SLI concentrations are normal or only marginally elevated, however, requires reliable provocative tests. Increased plasma SLI concentrations have been reported after intravenous infusion of tolbutamide and arginine, and decreased SLI concentrations have been observed after intravenous infusion of diazoxide. Arginine is a well-established stimulant for normal D cells and thus is unlikely to differentiate between normal and supranormal somatostatin secretion. The same may be true for diazoxide, which has been shown to decrease SLI secretion from normal dog pancreas as well as in patients with somatostatinoma. Tolbutamide stimulates SLI release from normal dog and rat pancreas, but no change was found in circulating SLI concentrations of three healthy human subjects after intravenous injection of 1 g of tolbutamide. Therefore, at present, tolbutamide appears to be a candidate for a provocative agent in the diagnosis of somatostatinoma, but its reliability must be established in a greater number of patients and controls. Until then, it may be necessary to measure plasma SLI concentrations during routine workups for postprandial dyspepsia and gallbladder disorders, for diabetes in patients without a family history, and for unexplained steatorrhea, because these findings can be early signs of somatostatinoma. Tolbutamide infusions are considered to have significant risks and should only be administered under strict medical observation.

IDC-9 CODE: Somatostatinoma (No Single Code; See Below for Individual Sites)

IDC-9 CODE: Malignant Neoplasm of the Pancreas, Producing Insulin, Somatostatin, and Glucagon
Islets of Langerhans 157.4

IDC-9 CODE: Malignant Neoplasm of the Intestine
Intestinal tract, part unspecified 159.0
Uncertain behavior, neoplasm of the intestine 235.2

IDC-9 CODE: Diabetes
Type 1 (not specified as uncontrolled) 250.01
Type 1 (uncontrolled) 250.03
Type 2 (or unspecified) 250.00
Type 2 (uncontrolled) 250.02
Hypoglycemia 250.8

ICD-9: CODE: Hypoglycemia 251.1

ICD-9 CODE: Reactive Hypoglycemia 251.2

IDC-9 CODE: Gallbladder Disease 575.9
Congenital 751.60

ICD-9 CODE: Diarrhea 787.91

ICD-9 CODE: Functional 564.5

ICD-9 CODE: Achlorhydria 536.0

IDC-9 CODE: Hypochlorhydria 536.8
Neurotic 306.4
Psychogenic 306.4

ICD-9 CODES for Primary Islet Cell Tumor Sites

Sites	Malignant	Benign	Uncertain Behavior	Unspecified
Ampulla	156.2	211.5	235.3	239.0
Duodenum	152.0	211.2	235.2	239.0
Jejunum	152.1	211.2	235.2	239.0
Pancreas	157.9	211.6	235.5	239.0
Body	157.1	211.6	235.5	239.0
Head	157.0	211.6	235.5	239.0
Islet cell	157.4	211.7	235.5	239.0
Neck	157.8	211.6	235.5	239.0
Tail	157.2	211.6	235.5	239.0

ICD-9 CODES for Metastatic Sites

Sites	Malignant
Supraclavicular	196.0
Abdominal	196.2
Mediastinal	196.1
Retroperitoneal	196.2
Liver	197.7
Bone	198.5
Lung	162.0
Brain	191.9

(See Somatostatin [Somatotropin Release–Inhibiting Factor (SRIF)] [Chapter 3] for specific tests and CPT codes)

PPOMA

Pancreatic polypeptide (PP) was discovered in 1972 by Chance and colleagues. These authors discovered and purified a single protein peak from a crude insulin preparation. In mammals, 93% of the cells producing PP are located in the pancreas. Meal ingestion, cerebral stimulation, and hormone administration have dramatic effects on circulating levels of PP. A biologic role for PP has not been established, however.

WHAT TO LOOK FOR

Distinguishing Signs and Symptoms

The only physiologic effects of PP that are recognized in humans are the inhibition of gallbladder contraction and pancreatic enzyme secretion. Thus, a tumor deriving from PP cells is expected to be clinically silent, although this is not always the case. For example, a tumor that invaded the bile ducts producing biliary obstruction was found to be a PPoma. It has been suggested that WDHHA, which is seen in GEP endocrine tumors, may have its origin in PP overproduction. The picture is complicated by the fact that mixed tumors, PP-cell hyperplasia in association with other functioning islet cell tumors, ductal hyperplasia of PP cells, nesidioblastosis, and multiple islet tumors producing PP also have been described, either alone or as part of the MEN-I syndrome **(Table 1-5)**.

Table 1-5. Coincident Elevations of Pancreatic Polypeptide

Tumor Type	Proportion of Patients With Coincident Elevations	Pancreatic Polypeptide Level in Plasma (pg/mL) or Other Laboratory Abnormalities
Endocrine-secreting tumors	22%<en>77%	>1000
Carcinoid tumors	29%<en>50%	>1000
Adenocarcinomas	53 patients	Not elevated
Nonfunctional GEP tumors	50%<en>75%	Slightly raised
Nonfunctional GEP tumors	50%<en>75%	Secretin more elevated

A response of greater than 5000 pg/min/mL (i.e., integrated response) is more than two standard deviations (SD) above that observed in healthy persons. In the absence of factors, such as chronic renal failure, that are known to cause marked elevation of PP levels, a markedly elevated PP level in an older, healthy patient occasionally may indicate a nonfunctioning pancreatic endocrine tumor. Differentiation of a high basal concentration in a healthy person from that appearing in patients with tumor is difficult. It has been suggested that administration of atropine would suppress PP concentrations in healthy subjects and would fail to do so in patients with tumors, but this has not been subjected to extensive examination.

ICD-9 CODE: PPoma (No Single Code; See Below for Individual Sites)

ICD-9 CODES for Primary Islet Cell Tumor Sites

Sites	Malignant	Benign	Uncertain Behavior	Unspecified
Ampulla	156.2	211.5	235.3	239.0
Duodenum	152.0	211.2	235.2	239.0
Jejunum	152.1	211.2	235.2	239.0
Pancreas	157.9	211.6	235.5	239.0
Body	157.1	211.6	235.5	239.0
Head	157.0	211.6	235.5	239.0
Islet cell	157.4	211.7	235.5	239.0
Neck	157.8	211.6	235.5	239.0
Tail	157.2	211.6	235.5	239.0

ICD-9 CODES for Metastatic Sites

Sites	Malignant
Supraclavicular	196.0
Abdominal	196.2
Mediastinal	196.1
Retroperitoneal	196.2
Liver	197.7
Bone	198.5
Lung	162.0
Brain	191.9

(See Pancreatic Polypeptide [PP] [Chapter 3] and Meal [Sham Feeding] Stimulation for Vagal Integrity [Chapter 5] for specific tests and CPT codes)

Reference

1. Gepts W, de Mey J. [Pancreatic polypeptide.] [Article in French.] Diabetes Metab. Dec;4(4):275-83, 1978.

Ghrelinoma

Since its recent discovery, there have been about 650 publications on this peptide, indicating a profound interest in the newest GEP hormone capable of stimulating growth hormone (GH) release by activation of the GH secretogogue type 1a (GHS-R1a) receptor. Ghrelin is the first natural hormone in which a hydroxyl group on one of its serine residues is acylated by n-octanoic acid. This acylation is essential for binding to the GHS-R1a receptor, for the GH-releasing capacity, and also likely for its other actions. Although it has been found to co-segregate with glucagon and insulin by some authors, this is not consistent, and most would agree that its cell of origin in the pancreas constitutes a new cell type.

Ghrelin stimulates the following:

- GH release in animals and humans by acting at both the pituitary and hypothalamic level
- Release of ACTH and prolactin, gastric acid secretion, and intestinal motility
- Gastric motility and gastric acid secretion

Ghrelin regulates the following:

- Energy balance
- Increased appetite and food intake
- Modulation of insulin secretion negatively
- Exertion of a tonic inhibitory role on insulin secretion in animals and humans
- Suppressed by hyperglycemia and insulin, and may, in addition, have a direct role on glycogenolysis

Ghrelin increases the following:

- Blood glucose levels
- Insulin resistance when administered systemically in humans

The expression of ghrelin protein and/or mRNA has recently been identified in almost all gastric and intestinal carcinoids as well as pancreatic NETs. There have been two case reports of ghrelinomas: in one, ghrelin was co-secreted with glucagon in a predominantly glucagon expression syndrome, whereas in the other nonfunctioning tumor, ghrelin levels were greater than 12,000 pM (normal, 300 pM). Despite the 50-fold increase in ghrelin levels, the patient had normal serum GH and insulin-like growth factor type 1 (IGF-1) levels. In this study no attempt was made to distinguish acylated ghrelin from the nonacylated variety, thus all the circulating ghrelin may have indeed been biologically inert.

Based on the physiologic effects of ghrelin, one would expect that the clinical features of a ghrelinoma would include the following:

- Hyperglycemia
- Insulin deficiency
- Insulin resistance
- GH excess
- Increased IGF-1 levels,
- Acromegaly
- Gastric acid hypersecretion
- Intestinal dysmotility

What to Look For

Distinguishing Signs and Symptoms

Ghrelin is a 28–amino acid acylated peptide related to the oxyntomodulin family of intestinal peptides. This peptide was isolated from the X/A-like neuroendocrine cells of the rat and human stomach. It is predominantly produced by the stomach but is also detectable in many other tissues:

- Bowel
- Hypothalamus
- Pituitary
- Pancreas
- Co-segregating with pancreatic alpha cells
- Possibly with pancreatic beta cells

Hormones and Peptides

- Ghrelin
- IGF-1
- CGA

Diagnosis

It seems for now that ghrelin is another hormone produced in almost all GEP NETs; has little, if any, biologic activity; and may be useful as a marker for response to therapy. In terms of screening, ghrelin does not seem to offer a great deal over conventional markers. However, in time it may demonstrate an ability to predict tumors. The initial excitement regarding ghrelin may run a parallel course with the excitement related to the discovery of PP; like PP, ghrelin has since been found to be a nonspecific marker because of its lack of a biologic effect. The difference is that ghrelin has been shown to have many effects when administered in the acylated form, and the increase in the endogenous levels of ghrelin in these tumors may be a variant of the acylated form without biologic activity. This peptide may, however, retain sufficient structural epitopes to be recognized by the antisera to ghrelin. Acylation-specific antisera will help to resolve part of this question.

ICD-9 CODE: Hyperglycemia 790.6

ICD-9 CODE: Diabetes Type I (Insulin Deficiency)

Not stated as uncontrolled 250.01
Uncontrolled 250.03

ICD-9 CODE: Dysmetabolic Syndrome X (Insulin Resistance) 277.7

ICD-9 CODE: Acromegaly 253.0

ICD-9 CODE: Gastric Acid Hypersecretion 536.8

ICD-9 CODE: Diarrhea (Intestinal Dysmotility) 787.91

ICD-9 CODE: Carcinoid Syndrome 259.2

ICD-9 CODES for Primary Islet Cell Tumor Sites

Sites	Malignant	Benign	Uncertain Behavior	Unspecified
Ampulla	156.2	211.5	235.3	239.0
Duodenum	152.0	211.2	235.2	239.0
Jejunum	152.1	211.2	235.2	239.0
Pancreas	157.9	211.6	235.5	239.0
Body	157.1	211.6	235.5	239.0
Head	157.0	211.6	235.5	239.0
Islet cell	157.4	211.7	235.5	239.0
Neck	157.8	211.6	235.5	239.0
Tail	157.2	211.6	235.5	239.0

ICD-9 CODES for Islet Cell Tumor Metastatic Sites

Sites	Malignant
Supraclavicular	196.0
Abdominal	196.2
Mediastinal	196.1
Retroperitoneal	196.2
Liver	197.7
Bone	198.5
Lung	162.0
Brain	191.9

(See Oral Glucose Tolerance Test for Diabetes, Insulinoma, Impaired Glucose Tolerance, Metabolic Syndrome, PCOS, Reactive Hypoglycemia, and Acromegaly [Chapter 5], MEN Syndrome Screen [Chapter 4], and GI–Neuroendocrine Tests [Chapter 4] for specific tests and CPT codes)

MULTIPLE ENDOCRINE NEOPLASIA SYNDROMES

Multiple endocrine neoplasia type I (MEN-I) involves the following:

- Pituitary gland
- Pancreas
- Parathyroid glands

The pituitary tumors are primarily prolactinomas, the pancreatic tumors are PPomas, and the gastrinomas, with rare instances of insulinoma, are more commonly nesidioblastosis or hyperplasia of beta cells and parathyroid hyperplasia rather than adenoma. These tumors are associated with the loss of a tumor suppressor gene on chromosome 11q13. This is the same chromosome on which the insulin gene has been located. It has been suggested, but not proven, that allelic losses in the MEN-I tumor suppressor gene located in the 11q13 region also might be responsible for sporadic parathyroid and pituitary tumors as well as NETs of the stomach, pancreas, and intestine. The few cases of carcinoid tumors studied have not shown losses in the 11q13 region.

Multiple endocrine neoplasia type IIa (MEN-IIa) syndrome is characterized by the occurrence of the following tumors:

- Pheochromocytomas
- Medullary carcinoma of the thyroid (MCT)
- Parathyroid hyperplasia

Multiple endocrine neoplasia type IIb (MEN-IIb), has stigmata of cutaneous and mucosal neuromas and is not associated with parathyroid hyperplasia. MEN-IIa and MEN-IIb and familial MCT are associated with mutations of the RET protooncogene, which is a conventional dominant oncogene located on 10q11.2. Although mutations in this region have been associated with sporadic MCT, the role, if any, of this gene in sporadic GEP tumors is not known. Occasionally there are crossover syndromes in which features of one syndrome occur in the milieu of the other syndrome (e.g., pheochromocytomas appearing in MEN-I).

Diagnosis

Diagnostic tests for the following:

- MCT
- Calcitonin
- Calcium infusion
- RET protooncogene
- Pheochromocytoma
- Vanillyl mandelic acid (VMA), epinephrine, norepinephrine
- Glucagon stimulation
- ^{131}I-MIBG

ICD-9 CODE: Malignant Neoplasm of the Thyroid Gland 193

ICD-9 CODE: Polyglandular Activity in Multiple Endocrine Adenomatosis 258.0

ICD-9 CODE: Pheochromocytoma (M8700/0)
Malignant (M8700/3)
Specified site–see Neoplasm by site, malignant
Unspecified site 194.0
Benign
Specified site–see Neoplasm by site, benign
Unspecified site 227.0
Uncertain behavior
Adrenal neoplasm 239.7
Neoplasm of bladder 239.4
Neoplasm of sympathetic nervous system 239.2

ICD-9 CODE: Medullary Carcinoma Thyroid (M8510/3)
With amyloid stroma (M8511/3)
Specified site, thyroid 193
Unspecified site 193
With lymphoid stroma (M8512/3)
Malignant thyroid 193
Uncertain behavior, neoplasm of thyroid 237.4

ICD-9 CODE: Parathyroid Hyperplasia 252.01

ICD-9 CODES for Primary Islet Cell Tumor Sites

Site	Malignant	Benign	Uncertain Behavior	Unspecified
Pancreas	157.9	211.6	235.5	239.0
Body	157.1	211.6	235.5	239.0
Head	157.0	211.6	235.5	239.0
Islet cell	157.4	211.7	235.5	239.0
Neck	157.8	211.6	235.5	239.0
Tail	157.2	211.6	235.5	239.0
Pituitary gland	194.3	227.3	237.0	239.7
Parathyroid gland	194.1	227.1	237.4	239.7
Thyroid	193	226	237.4	239.7

ICD-9 CODES for Islet Cell Tumor Metastatic Sites

Sites	Malignant
Supraclavicular	196.0
Abdominal	196.2
Mediastinal	196.1
Retroperitoneal	196.2
Liver	197.7
Bone	198.5
Lung	162.0
Brain	191.9

(See MEN Syndrome Screen [Chapter 4] for specific tests and CPT codes)

NEUROENDOCRINE TUMORS IN CHILDREN

The vast majority of NETs in children are similar to their adult counterparts with the exception of the neuroblastoma, which is unique to infancy and is an aggressive tumor.

CARCINOID

Carcinoid tumors may be the most common NET in childhood. Nearly 15% of carcinoid tumors are found in patients under the age of 25 years. The most common site of carcinoid in children is the appendix, and it often is an incidental finding. Carcinoid may be recognized in adolescents only when it metastasizes. Flushing and diarrhea are common symptoms in healthy children, which makes the diagnosis of carcinoid more difficult.

NEUROBLASTOMA

This tumor may be the second most common NET of childhood, and usually it presents as a mass. It also can present with diarrhea if tumor cells produce VIP. CGA and neuropeptide Y (NPY) levels in blood are helpful for assessing the extent of disease and should be obtained simultaneously with VIP levels. Hypertension also may be seen if catecholamine synthesis is high. Twenty-four–hour urine VMA (and homovanillic acid [HVA]) levels are important screening tests in all neuroblastomas, whether or not hypertension is present. OctreoScan® or ^{131}I-MIBG scan also can be helpful in evaluating extent of disease and may be diagnostic. Biopsy of lymph node, bone marrow, or primary lesion is necessary to confirm the diagnosis.

GASTRINOMA

Diarrhea and peptic ulcer disease are common in children. Gastrinoma is extremely rare in children, but has reported as early as 7 years of age. Normal gastrin levels are similar in children and adults; thus, measuring fasting gastrin levels is an easy and extremely useful test in diagnosing this condition. However, chronic use of PPI can raise gastrin levels, therefore these drugs should be discontinued for at least 72 hours before obtaining blood for measurement of gastrin levels. Note that gastrin levels may remain elevated for several months after discontinuing PPI.

INSULINOMA/NESIDIOBLASTOSIS

Nesidioblastosis is the result of an overactive pancreas and most often presents at birth with hypoglycemia unresponsive to feeding or intravenous glucose. Neonatal nesidioblastosis, like adult-onset nesidioblastosis, is characterized by islet cell hyperplasia. These hyperplastic islets often vary widely in size. This condition often resolves with close follow-up and octreotide therapy but may resurface when these children reach puberty. Surgical intervention is rarely required. In cases requiring surgery, a subtotal pancreatectomy may be lifesaving. Insulin and C-peptide levels are measured in blood, and normal levels are similar to those in adults. Some of these tumors may be caused by mutations in the sulfonylurea receptor.

Multiple Endocrine Neoplasia

Multiple endocrine neoplasia type I presents in parathyroid, pancreas, and pituitary glands. A family history of MEN-I should prompt genetic screening for all members. MEN-IIa occurs in parathyroid, thyroid, MCT, and adrenal glands (pheochromocytoma), whereas MEN-IIb occurs in MCT, pheochromocytoma, and neural tumors. Family history and blood pressure measurements are the most important screening tools. Children can be tested and a diagnosis made as early as 4 years of age using blood calcitonin levels; the pentagastrin stimulation test, although still available, has now been replaced by genetic screening for the RET protooncogene. Urine catecholamines are also important markers and can be determined using a 24-hour urine test.

Pheochromocytoma

Pheochromocytoma is associated with MEN-IIa and -IIb, von Hippel-Lindau (VHL) syndrome, and neurofibromatosis. The peak incidence occurs between 9 and 12 years of age, nearly 10% of all pheochromocytomas occur in children, and 10% of these are malignant. Headaches, palpitations, diaphoresis, and hypertension are the most common symptoms. Diagnostic testing should include 24-hour urine test for creatinine, VMA, catecholamines, and metanephrine as well as plasma levels of metanephrine and CGA. Since pheochromocytomas can be seen in adolescents and young adults, drug interference with metanephrine testing should be ruled out with a careful history of medication and illicit drug use. False-positive metanephrine tests can be caused by buspirone, benzodiazepines, methyldopa, labetalol, tricyclic antidepressants; levodopa, ethanol, amphetamines, sotalol, and chlorpromazine.

Extra-adrenal pheochromocytomas comprise nearly 25% of pheochromocytomas in children and are characteristic of VHL syndrome. Symptoms are the same as for pheochromocytoma.

Pheochromocytoma is associated with MEN-IIa and -IIb, VHL, and neurofibromatosis. The peak incidence occurs between 9 and 12 years of age, and nearly 10% of all pheochromocytomas occur in children and 10% of these are malignant. Headaches, palpitations, diaphoresis, and hypertension are the most common symptoms. Diagnostic testing should include 24-hour urine for creatinine, VMA, catecholamines and metanephrine and plasma metanephrine and CGA. Since pheochromocytomas can be seen in adolescents and young adults, drug interference with metanephrine testing should be ruled out with a careful history of medication and illicit use. False-positive metanephrines can be caused by buspirone, benzodiazepines, methyldopa, labetalol, tricyclic antidepressants, levodopa, ethanol, amphetamines, sotalol, and chlorpromazine.

Paraganglioma

Extra-adrenal pheochromocytomas comprise nearly 25% of pheochromocytomas in children and are characteristic of VHL syndrome. Symptoms are the same as for pheochromocytoma.

Munchausen's by Proxy

Diarrhea, flushing, sweating, and fatigue are hallmark symptoms of neuroendocrine (carcinoid) tumors; however, each of these symptoms is common in otherwise healthy children and also can be associated with viral infections, topical exposures, and allergies. A parent, relative, or guardian can also easily induce this symptom complex. Diarrhea can be induced with laxatives, and their administration should be ascertained in the screening process. Ricins cause overall irritation of the GI tract, and castor oil induces vomiting as well as some GI upset. These "medicines" can be measured in the stool, and pH and stool electrolytes determined to elucidate their presence.

Flushing is seldom witnessed by medical personnel. It can be caused by allergic reactions, selective serotonin uptake inhibitors such as Zoloft or Prozac, and even by overuse of vitamin A.

Sweating is likewise difficult to provoke in an office setting and thus is seldom witnessed by medical personnel. The sweating associated with Hodgkin's Disease—described as "drenching"—most often occurs at night. This sweating is easily distinguished from that caused by NETs.

Fatigue is a "soft" symptom that is very difficult to evaluate but is most often the result of too little sleep. Children and adolescents should have 8 to 10 hours of sleep each night—significantly more than most adults require.

Those patients with overly solicitous parents who are extremely knowledgeable about medical terminology and procedures and those patients with a history of multiple professional caregivers should raise the possibility of Munchausen's by proxy in the differential diagnosis. The availability of medical information on the internet has contributed to this explosion of medical knowledge among lay persons, but in the case of Munchausen's, important details may be missing from the child's history that rule against NETs as the true cause of the symptoms.

ICD-9 CODE: Pheochromocytoma (M8700/0)

- Malignant (M8700/3)
  - Specified site–see Neoplasm by site, malignant
  - Unspecified site 194.0
- Benign
  - Specified site–see Neoplasm by site, benign
  - Unspecified site 227.0
- Uncertain behavior
  - Adrenal neoplasm 239.7
  - Neoplasm of bladder 239.4
  - Neoplasm of sympathetic nervous system 239.2

ICD-9 CODE: Insulinoma (M8151/0)

- Malignant (M8151/3)
  - Pancreas 157.4

Unspecified site 157.4
Specified site–see Neoplasm by site, malignant
Benign, unspecified site 211.7
Uncertain behavior, neoplasm of pancreas 235.5

ICD-9 CODE: Gastrinoma (M8153/1)
Malignant (M8153/3)
Pancreas 157.4
Specified site–see Neoplasm by site, malignant
Unspecified site 157.4
Specified site–see Neoplasm by site, uncertain behavior
Benign, unspecified site 235.5
Uncertain behavior, neoplasm of pancreas 235.5

ICD-9 CODE: Neuroblastoma (M9500/3)
Olfactory (M9522/3) 160
Specified site–see Neoplasm by site, malignant
Unspecified site 194.0
Uncertain behavior, olfactory neoplasm 237.9

ICD-9 CODE: Carcinoid Syndrome 259.2

ICD-9 CODE: MEN-I and -II 258.0

For additional ICD-9 codes, please see the sections on specific NETs. Codes for children are the same as adults.

(See MEN Syndrome Screen [Chapter 4], Chromogranin A [CGA] [Chapter 3], and Flushing Syndrome Tests [Chapter 4] for specific tests and CPT codes)

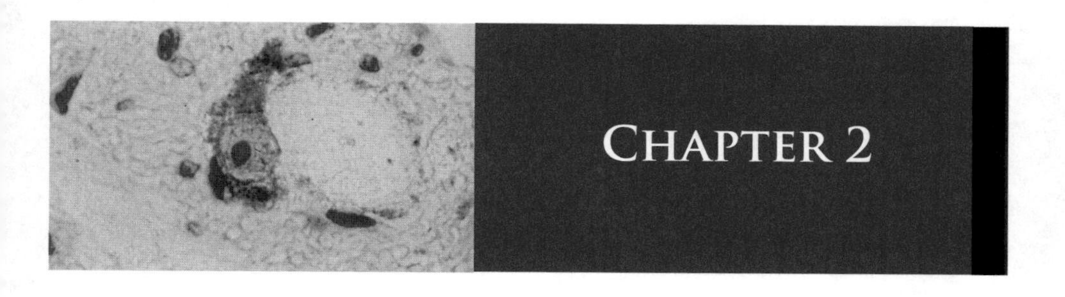

CHAPTER 2

CLINICAL PRESENTATIONS AND THEIR SYNDROMES, INCLUDING ICD-9 CODES

The frequency of clinical manifestations related to the GEP neuroendocrine system, is as follows:

Flushing	84%
Diarrhea	79%
Heart disease	37%
Bronchoconstriction	17%
Myopathy	7%
Pigmentation	5%
Arthropathy	5%
Hyper-hypoglycemia	<1%
Ulcer disease	<1%
Dermopathy	<1%

Flushing

Flushing, a cardinal symptom of carcinoid tumors, occurs in a variety of other conditions. A good rule of thumb is if the flushing is "wet" (accompanied by sweating), it is due to a cause other than carcinoid. **Table 2-1** lists the differential diagnosis and the features that help distinguish flushing caused by carcinoid from flushing associated with other conditions.

Table 2-1. Features Associated With Various Flushing Syndromes

Flushing Syndrome	Associated Features
Carcinoid	Diarrhea, wheezing
MCT	Mass in neck, family history
Pheochromocytoma	Paroxysmal hypertension, tachycardia
Diabetes	Autonomic neuropathy/chlorpropamide
Menopause	Cessation of menses
Autonomic epilepsy	Diencephalic seizures
Panic syndrome	Phobias, anxiety
Mastocytosis	Dyspepsia, peptic ulcer, dermatographia
Drugs	Niacin, alcohol, calcium channel blockers
Idiopathic	Diagnosis by exclusion
Cardiac	Angina in women, mitral valve prolapse

What to Look For

Distinguishing Signs and Symptoms

There are two varieties of flushing in carcinoid syndrome:

1. Midgut carcinoid: The flush usually is faint pink to red in color and involves the face and upper trunk as far as the nipple line. The flush is initially provoked by alcohol and food containing tyramine (e.g., blue cheese, chocolate, aged or cured sausage, red wine). With time, the flush may occur spontaneously and without provocation. It usually lasts only a few minutes and may occur many times per day. It generally does not leave permanent discoloration.
2. Foregut tumors: The flush often is more intense, of longer duration, and purplish in hue. It is frequently followed by telangiectasia and involves not only the upper trunk but may also affect the limbs. The limbs may become acrocyanotic, and the appearance of the nose resembles that of rhinophyma. The skin of the face often thickens, and assumes leonine facies resembling that seen in leprosy and acromegaly.

THE NEXT STEP

Other Clinical Conditions

Because flushing cannot always be attributed to carcinoid syndrome, as mentioned previously, the differential diagnosis of flushing is extremely important and includes the following:

- Postmenopausal state
- Simultaneous ingestion of chlorpropamide and alcohol
- Panic attacks
- MCT
- Autonomic epilepsy
- Autonomic neuropathy
- Mastocytosis
- Ganglioneuromas
- Carotid body tumors
- Pheochromocytomas

Hormones and Peptides

Measure the levels of the following hormones and peptides ascribed to flushing in carcinoid syndrome:

- Prostaglandins
- Kinins
- Serotonin (5-HT)
- Vasoactive neuropeptides (serotonin, dopamine, histamine)
- 5-HIAA
- Substance P
- Neurotensin
- Somatostatin
- Motilin
- VIP
- Neuropeptide K
- Gastrin-releasing peptide (GRP)

Several tests are used to identify the cause of flushing in carcinoid syndrome **(Table 2-2)**.

Table 2-2. Tests to Identify Cause of Flushing

Clinical Condition	Tests
Carcinoid	Urine 5-HIAA, 5-HTP, substance P, CGRP, CGA
MCT	Calcitonin, calcium infusion, RET protooncogene
Pheochromocytoma	VMA, epinephrine, norepinephrine, glucagon stimulation, ^{131}I-MIBG
Diabetic autonomic neuropathy	Heart rate variability, 2-hour PP, glucose
Menopause	FSH
Epilepsy	Electroencephalogram
Panic syndrome	Pentagastrin/ACTH
Mastocytosis	Plasma histamine, urine tryptase
Hypomastia, mitral prolapse	Cardiac echogram

ICD-9 CODE: Flushing 782.62

ICD-9 CODE: Carcinoid Syndrome 259.2

ICD-9 CODE: Medullary Carcinoma Thyroid (M8510/3)
- With amyloid stroma (M8511/3)
  - Specified site, thyroid 193
  - Unspecified site 193
- With lymphoid stroma (M8512/3)
  - Malignant thyroid 193

ICD-9 CODE: Pheochromocytoma (M8700/0)
- Malignant (M8700/3)
  - Specified site–see Neoplasm by site, malignant
  - Unspecified site 194.0
- Benign
  - Specified site–see Neoplasm by site, benign
  - Unspecified site 227.0

ICD-9 CODE: Diabetes, Autonomic Neuropathy 250.6

ICD-9 CODE: Autonomic Epilepsy
- Without mention of intractable epilepsy 345.50
- With intractable epilepsy 345.51

ICD-9 CODE: Panic Attack 300.01

ICD-9 CODE: Mastocytosis 753.33
- Malignant 202.6
- Systemic 202.6

ICD-9 CODE: Hypomastia (Congenital) 757.6

ICD-9 CODE: Mitral Prolapse 424.0

(See Flushing Syndrome Tests [Chapter 4] for specific tests and individual CPT codes)

DIARRHEA

Watery diarrhea syndrome (WDHHA), which is caused by a pancreatic islet cell tumor, was first identified by Verner and Morrison in 1958. As implied by its name, the primary characteristic is watery diarrhea. A critical distinguishing difference from ZE is the absence of hyperacidity and the marked presence of hypokalemia. Diarrhea of ZE improves with inhibition of acid secretion, whereas in WDHHA it does not. The WDHHA usually begins with intermittent diarrhea, but as the tumor grows, the episodic diarrhea becomes continuous and persists despite fasting (i.e., it is secretory, not malabsorptive). Hypercalcemia occurs in WDHHA because of direct effects of VIP on bone. It is important to differentiate this cause of hypercalcemia from the hypercalcemia caused by excess PTH release from parathyroid glands seen in the sporadic (usually caused by adenomas) or familial (usually the result of hyperplastic glands) forms of hyperthyroidism. Factitious diarrhea can be difficult to distinguish and requires the demonstration of an osmolar gap. If 2x $[Na^{+}+K^{+}]$ is less than stool osmolality (i.e., osmotic gap), search for idiogenic osmoles.

The following are characteristics of secretory diarrhea:

- Large-volume stools
- Persists during fasting
- 2 x $[Na^{+}+K^{+}]$ = stool osmolality

The following are characteristics of osmotic diarrhea:

- Small volume (<1 L/d)
- Disappears with fasting

WHAT TO LOOK FOR

Distinguishing Signs and Symptoms

- Profuse diarrhea with the appearance of weak tea
- Presence of marked hypokalemia and hyperchloremic acidosis
- Initial intermittent diarrhea, becoming continuous as tumor grows
- Secretory nature of diarrhea (i.e., does not disappear even after fasting for 48 hours)
- Absence of gastric hyperacidity (a major feature distinguishing WDHHA from ZE)
- Atrophic gastritis or pernicious anemia or gastric carcinoid type 1
- Hypochlorhydria resulting from the gastric inhibitory effect of VIP
- Secretion of HCO_3 and K^+ causes life-threatening loss of electrolytes into the stool
- Increased intestinal motility as well as secretion adding to the diarrhea
- Hypercalcemia not due to PTH or PTHRP
- Hyperglycemia or abnormal glucose tolerance
- Dilation of the gallbladder
- Flushing
- Weight loss
- Colic

THE NEXT STEP

Patients with watery diarrhea are often severely dehydrated, and their fluid balance and electrolytes should be corrected before specific diagnostic tests are initiated, except for evaluation of stool electrolytes and osmolarity.

Diagnostic tests should be selected to:

- Exclude atrophic gastritis, pernicious anemia, and gastric carcinoid
- Exclude use of proton pump inhibitors
- Exclude ZE
- Determine the probability of a pancreatic-based source of watery diarrhea (VIP, PP, MCT, CT, and OctreoScan®)
- Eliminate other syndromes masquerading as WDHHA and producing similar symptoms

Hormones and Peptides

Vasoactive intestinal polypeptide is the primary peptide produced by the majority of pancreatic tumors (VIPomas) causing WDHHA, but substance P, PP, calcitonin gene–related peptide (CGRP) and thyrocalcitonin (TCT) have also been implicated in NET-related diarrhea. Because VIP is also produced by neural cells, elevated levels of other GI and pancreatic hormones and peptides may be markers for establishing the presence of a pancreatic tumor associated with diarrhea. WDHHA in children is most commonly due to a nonpancreatic NET such as neuroblastoma. Occasionally, adults with pheochromocytomas may secrete VIP, which releases prolactin and is a vasodilator in the corpora cavernosa. However, this does not appear to be part of the clinical syndrome **(Fig. 2-1)**.

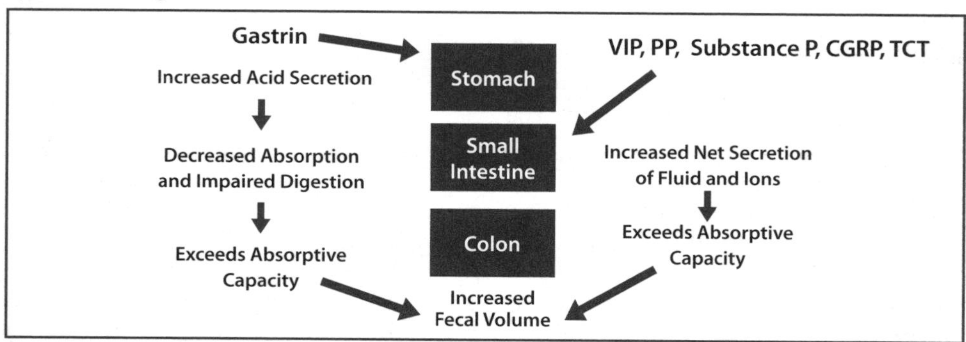

Figure 2-1. Pathogenesis of Endocrine Diarrhea

After mechanical causes have been ruled out, use the following ICD-9 codes:

ICD-9 CODE: Diarrhea 787.91

ICD-9 CODE: Functional 564.5

ICD-9 CODE: Achlorhydria 536.0

(See Table 1-1 for primary tumor sites and common metastatic tumor sites)
(See Diarrhea Syndrome Tests [Chapter 4] for specific tests and individual CPT codes)

Reference

1. Verner JV, Morrison AB. Islet cell tumor and a syndrome of refractory watery diarrhea and hypokalemia. *Am J Med.* Sept;25(3):374-80, 1958.

BRONCHOCONSTRICTION (WHEEZING)

Wheezing due to bronchospasm occurs in about one third of patients with carcinoid syndrome and in patients with mastocytosis.

WHAT TO LOOK FOR

Distinguishing Signs and Symptoms

Wheezing can be readily assessed at the bedside by asking the patient to breathe out as quickly as possible and listening to the trachea. Normally the wheezing is almost instantaneous, but with the expiratory bronchospasm in carcinoid and mastocytosis it is often prolonged. A test dose of octreotide acetate (100 μg) administered intravenously will relieve carcinoid bronchospasm. It is not known what effects octreotide has on asthma.

THE NEXT STEP

Lung function tests reveal a prolongation of forced expiratory volume in 1 second (FEV_1), which needs to be distinguished from asthma and chronic airways obstructive disease. Refer the patient to a pulmonologist.

Hormones and Peptides

Wheezing is predominantly the result of the bronchoconstrictive effects of substance P, histamine, and possibly 5-HT.

ICD-9 CODE: Wheezing 786.07

ICD-9 CODE: Bronchospasm 519.1

ICD-9 CODE: Carcinoid Syndrome 259.2

ICD-9 CODE: Asthma
Unspecified 493.90
With status asthmaticus 493.91
With (acute) exacerbation 493.92

(See Carcinoid Follow-Up Profile [Chapter 4] for individual tests and CPT codes for substance P, histamine, serotonin; see Bronchospasm Profile [Chapter 4] for specific tests and CPT codes)

DYSPEPSIA, PEPTIC ULCER

GASTRINOMA (ZOLLINGER-ELLISON SYNDROME)

Zollinger-Ellison syndrome is characterized by hyperacidity and gastrin hypersecretion from an islet cell tumor (gastrinoma) of the pancreas or duodenum. Approximately 90% of gastrinomas are found in the "gastrinoma" triangle, an area bordered by the confluence of the cystic and common ducts superiorly, the mesenteric vessels medially, and the lateral sweep of the "C" loop of the duodenum laterally. A primary gastrinoma is rarely found in the liver or ovary, and even more rarely in a lymph node. These tumors may be associated with peptic perforation, obstruction, hemorrhage, and/or hyperacidity. Atrophic gastritis, pernicious anemia, gastric carcinoid, chronic proton pump inhibitor use, and diabetic gastropathy may produce spuriously high gastrin levels. A high gastrin level in the absence of diarrhea suggests atrophic gastritis. Secretory diarrhea in the presence of achlorhydria with normal gastrin levels suggests a VIPoma. Gastric pH measurement remains a valuable tool in distinguishing the causes of hypergastrinemia. Even though this measurement is easily performed, it is often overlooked.

WHAT TO LOOK FOR

Distinguishing Signs and Symptoms

- Highly elevated level of gastrin
- Diarrhea that responds to PPI

THE NEXT STEP

In conjunction with gastric acid measurement, these syndromes may be distinguished, but provocative testing may be necessary.

Hormones and Peptides

Normal values of gastrin are 100 to 120 pg/mL. PPI will raise levels to 400 to 500 pg/mL. Fasting gastrin concentrations greater than 500 pg/mL in the presence of normal or excess gastric acid is suspicious of gastrinoma. Very high levels of greater than 1000 pg/mL may be pathognomic of gastrinoma. Pernicious anemia and atrophic gastritis can produce gastrin levels greater than 1000 pg/mL, which should alert the clinician to the possibility of gastric carcinoid. Endoscopic pH measurements are essential to distinguish ZE from atrophic gastritis, type 1 gastric carcinoid, and pernicious anemia.

ICD-9 CODE: Dyspepsia/Peptic Ulcer 536.8

ICD-9 CODE: Peptic Ulcer

Without obstruction 533.90
With obstruction 533.91
With hemorrhage 533.4
    Without obstruction 533.40
    With obstruction 533.1
    And perforation 533.6

Perforation (chronic) 533.5
With hemorrhage 533.6

ICD-9 CODE: Zollinger-Ellison/Gastrinoma 251.5
Malignant
Pancreas 157.4
Specified site–see Neoplasm by site, malignant
Unspecified site 157.4
Benign
Unspecified site 235.5
Uncertain behavior, see Neoplasm

(See Table 1-1 for primary tumor sites and common metastatic tumor sites)
(See Gastrin Test [Chapter 3] for specific tests and CPT codes)

HYPOGLYCEMIA

Hypoglycemia is a multifactorial disorder. Although the diagnosis of an insulin-secreting lesion of the pancreas is essential to successful management, it is critically important to rule out other causes of hypoglycemia.

WHAT TO LOOK FOR

Distinguishing Signs and Symptoms

- Organic hyperinsulinemia
  - Islet cell adenoma, carcinoma, hyperplasia, nesidioblastosis
- Fasting hypoglycemia
- Autoimmune with insulin antibodies
- Counter-regulatory hormone deficiency
  - Anterior pituitary insufficiency—GH, ACTH
  - Adrenocortical insufficiency
  - Severe hypothyroidism
  - Large nonislet tumor
  - Impaired hepatic function
  - Hepatocellular insufficiency
  - Ethanol/malnutrition
  - Sepsis
  - Specific enzymatic defects (childhood)
  - Impaired renal function
  - Substrate deficiency
  - Fanconi syndrome (renal loss)
  - Nursing
  - Severe inanition
  - Severe exercise
- Drug induced
  - Reactive hypoglycemia
  - Alimentary
  - "Pre-diabetes"
  - Endocrine
  - Idiopathic
- Factitious
  - Surreptitious insulin administration
  - Surreptitious sulfonylurea administration
  - Leukemoid reaction polycythemia
  - ACTH or GH administration
- Hyperinsulinemia
  - An accurate diagnosis of organic hyperinsulinemia can be established in most cases by a process of exclusion. The diagnosis can usually be made before extensive exploration of neoplastic causes.

- Autoimmunity
  - Syndromes of autoimmunity may lead to hypoglycemia. Antireceptor antibodies usually occur in the presence of other autoimmune disease, mimicking the effect of insulin and reducing insulin clearance. Insulin levels may be normal or high, but C-peptide levels are low because islet cells are suppressed.
- Reactive hypoglycemia
  - Autoimmune hypoglycemic disease syndrome usually occurs in the presence of other autoimmune disorders (e.g., Graves' disease, rheumatoid arthritis, lupus) and commonly produces reactive hypoglycemia from prolongation of the half-life of circulating insulin. This is also an important mechanism in late dumping syndrome. Insulin levels are generally extremely elevated, which may result from interference by antibodies with the particular insulin assay. C-peptide levels are usually low.
- Neoplasms
  - In the case of large mesenchymal neoplasms, the offending agent may be IGF-2; neither the size of the tumor nor the glucose metabolized by the tumor causes hyperglycemia; however, there is increased disposal of glucose by the liver mimicking the actions of insulin.
- Counter-regulatory hormone deficiency
  - Hypoglycemia resulting from conditions in which there is failure of gluconeogenesis or hormonal counter-regulations for (e.g. Addison's disease), hypopituitarism usually can be recognized clinically.
- Factitious hypoglycemia
  - Factitious hypoglycemia is extremely difficult to discern. If the patient uses insulin, there may be a low level of C-peptide, but if a sulfonylureas is being used, then insulin and C-peptide may be elevated. In this case look for the presence of insulin antibodies and sulfonylureas.

Non–Islet Cell Neoplasms Associated With Hypoglycemia

- Mesenchymal
  - Mesothelioma
  - Fibrosarcoma
  - Rhabdomyosarcoma
  - Leiomyosarcoma
  - Hemangiopericytoma
- Carcinoma
  - Hepatic: hepatoma, biliary carcinoma
  - Adrenocortical carcinoma
  - Genitourinary: hypernephroma, Wilms' tumor of the prostate
  - Reproductive: cervical or breast carcinoma
- Neurologic/neuroendocrine
  - Pheochromocytoma
  - Carcinoid
  - Neurofibroma

- Hematologic
  - Leukemia
  - Lymphoma
  - Myeloma

THE NEXT STEP

Hormones, Peptides, and Enzymes

- Insulin
- IGF-2
- C-peptide
- Glucagon-like peptide type 1 (GLP-1) and GIP
- Sulfonylurea
- ACTH
- GH
- Insulin antibodies
- Liver enzymes

ICD-9 CODE: Hypoglycemia 251
Diabetic 250.8
Due to insulin 251.0
Reactive 251.2

ICD-9 CODE: Hyperinsulinemia 251.2
NEC 51.1

ICD-9 CODE: Dumping Syndrome
Nonsurgical 536.8
Postgastrectomy 654.2

ICD-9 CODE: Complications of Drug Injection or Therapy 999.9

ICD-9 CODE: Complication of Surgical Procedure 998.9

(See Table 1-1 for primary tumor sites and common metastatic tumor sites)
(See Hypoglycemia/Insulinoma Screening Test [Chapter 4] for specific tests and CPT codes)

Dermopathy

When dermopathy occurs with glucagonoma syndrome it is also known by the acronym 4D, which stands for dermatosis, diarrhea, DVT, and depression. Pellagra-like eruptions occur in carcinoid as a result of niacin deficiency, and increased pigmentation occurs with MSH overproduction.

What to Look For

Distinguishing Signs and Symptoms

- Characteristic NME rash (82%)
- Pellagra rash forming a necklace and forearm pigmentation with the appearance of tiling
- Increased pigmentation in sun-exposed areas with overproduction of MSH
- Painful glossitis, angular stomatitis
- Normochromic normocytic anemia (61%)
- Weight loss (90%)
- Mild diabetes mellitus (80%)
- Hypoaminoacidemia
- DVT (50%)
- Depression (50%)

The Next Step

Hormones, Peptides, and Amino Acids

- Glucagon
- Plasma amino acids (tryptophan)
- α-MSH
- Serotonin
- 5-HIAA
- Niacin

ICD-9 CODE: Glucagonoma (M8152/0)—For Glucagonoma Rash

Malignant (M8152/3)

Pancreas 157.4

Unspecified site 157.4

Specified site–see Neoplasm by site, malignant

Benign

Specified site–see Neoplasm by site, benign

Unspecified site 211.7

Uncertain behavior, neoplasm of pancreas 235.5

ICD-9 CODE: Pellagra 265.2

(See Table 1-1 for primary tumor sites and common metastatic tumor sites)
(See Glucagon [Chapter 3] and Serotonin [Chapter 3] for specific tests and CPT codes)

Dumping Syndrome

Postgastrectomy dumping syndrome occurs in as many as 25% of patients undergoing ablative or bypass surgery on the pylorus. Approximately 5% of patients have debilitating dumping syndrome following major gastric resections. There may be varying degrees of this pathophysiologic state. Ingestion of cold or carbohydrate-rich foods may precipitate early dumping with cardiovascular (tachycardia and shock-like symptoms) and gastrointestinal components (explosive diarrhea and cramping). Classically, patients with dumping syndrome do not have symptoms with every meal; therefore they commonly use medication to control this syndrome only when they know that they are going to ingest foods that will provoke an attack. Late dumping is characterized by hypoglycemic events. These features can be explained by insulin-induced hypoglycemia. Alterations in gut peptide levels have been implicated in both early and late dumping syndromes. PP, glucagon, insulin, and motilin have been implicated in the pathogenesis of dumping syndrome.

What to Look For

Distinguishing Signs and Symptoms

Early Dumping Syndrome

Early dumping is caused by rapid shifts of water and electrolytes into the duodenum and proximal small bowel lumen in response to the introduction of hyperosmolar chyme into these regions. Fluid shifts into the gut lumen produce intravascular volume reduction, subsequent hemoconcentration, and an adrenergic shock-like response, producing the following symptoms:

- Diaphoresis
- Syncope
- Tachycardia
- Hypotension
- Borborygmus
- Explosive diarrhea

Late Dumping Syndrome

- Tremors
- Diaphoresis
- Syncope
- Mental confusion

The Next Step

Carbohydrate Test

Use a high-carbohydrate test meal to provoke dumping syndrome in a controlled clinical environment. This test meal contains 750 kcal, 21g protein, 30 g fat, and 99 g of carbohydrate (i.e., 2 eggs, 2 strips of bacon, a cup of decaffeinated coffee, 2 pieces of toast, 1 scoop of ice cream, and 1 ounce of chocolate syrup). The meal must be consumed within 10 minutes. Patients with dumping syndrome usually respond with significant rises in PP, insulin, and glucagon levels within 45 minutes of ingestion of this meal. Increases in motilin levels are usually seen 120 to 180 minutes after ingestion of a provocative meal.

Hormones and Peptides

- Insulin
- PP
- Glucagon
- GIP
- GLP-1
- Motilin

Octreotide Suppression Test

Octreotide acetate administration at low doses (100 µg 1 hour before meals) has been effectively used to control the symptoms of early dumping but is less efficacious in the control of late dumping. It can however, be used as a test of hormone and symptom responsiveness. Use of octreotide in patients with late dumping syndrome can be associated with worsening of hypoglycemia and should be done only in a controlled clinical environment.

ICD-9 CODE: Dumping Syndrome
Nonsurgical 536.8
Postgastrectomy 654.2

(See Table 1-1 for primary tumor sites and common metastatic tumor sites)
(See Provocative Test for Dumping Syndrome [Chapter 5] for further test instructions and CPT codes for specific hormone and peptide measurements)

Pancreatic Exocrine Diseases

Pancreatic exocrine diseases are not commonly associated with NETs. However, many of the neuroendocrine secretions are affected by neoplastic and non-neoplastic conditions. Additionally, therapeutic interventions used in the treatment of NETs may affect exocrine secretion.

The pancreas is an integrated organ of both endocrine and exocrine functions. The exocrine pancreas is composed of enzyme-secreting acini and the bicarbonate/fluid-secreting ductal system. Inflammatory and neoplastic diseases constitute some of the most prevalent and life-threatening diseases affecting the US population. Acute and chronic pancreatitis affects more than 200,000 individuals; although it often runs a mild course, up to 30% of cases are associated with significant morbidity and mortality. Meanwhile, more than 30,000 individuals are diagnosed with pancreatic cancer each year, with a 5-year survival rate of less than 10%. Recently, diagnostic imaging (CT, ultrasound [regular or endocscopic], and MRI) coupled with laboratory biomarkers have been used routinely for diagnosis of the pancreatic diseases.

What to Look For

Distinguishing Signs and Symptoms

Acute Pancreatitis

- Abdominal pain with elevated pancreatic enzymes (amylase, lipas, and trypsin) in blood and/or urine.
- Clinical manifestation may range from mild and self-limited abdominal discomfort to acute abdomen with shock.

Laboratory Diagnosis of Acute Pancreatitis. Serum amylase and lipase levels are widely and routinely used for the diagnosis of acute pancreatitis clinically. However, the prognostic capability of both of these enzymes to determine the severity of disease has been poor.

The Next Step

The following guidelines **(Table 2-3)** are suggested based on the recent evidence available for various biochemical markers to distinguish between mild and severe acute pancreatitis in early stages and during the clinical course of the disease.

Table 2-3. Assessment of Severity of Acute Pancreatitis

- At the time of admission
  - IL-6: ELISA (cutoff value 400 pg/mL)
  - IL-8: ELISA (cutoff value >400 pg/mL)
  - IL-10: ELISA (cutoff value >100 pg/mL)
  - APACHE II: Score greater than 7
- First 24 hours of hospitalization
  - Urine trypsinogen activation peptide: ELISA (cutoff value >35 nmol/L)
  - Urine Trypsinogen-2: dipstick (cutoff value >2000 μg/L)
  - Polymorphonuclear release: ELISA (cutoff value >300 μg/L)
- First 48 hours of hospitalization
  - C-reactive protein: automated (cutoff value > 150 mg/L)
  - APACHE score: >3
- Tools that require further validation
  - Cytokines
    - IL-1
    - TNFα, TNFβ, TNFα receptor
  - Pancreatic markers
    - Carboxypeptidase B activation peptide

WHAT TO LOOK FOR

Distinguishing Signs and Symptoms

Chronic Pancreatitis

Alcohol abuse is one of the leading causes of chronic pancreatitis. This condition is characterized by a long interval between the onset of alcohol abuse and onset of symptoms, which include the following:

- Recurrent upper abdominal pain
- Weight loss
- Diarrhea
- Steatorrhea with or without endocrine insufficiency (diabetes)
- Pancreatic calcification

Laboratory Diagnosis of Chronic Pancreatitis. Pancreatic serum enzymes such as amylase and lipase are elevated only during the acute attack, but remain normal during symptom-free intervals. Moreover, as the disease progresses, serum pancreatic enzymes are no longer elevated because of pancreatic parenchymal damages accompanied by exocrine pancreatic insufficiency.

The Next Step

To diagnose chronic pancreatitis, imagining procedures (US, CT, or endoscopic ultrasound) and pancreatic function tests should be combined.

Hormones, Peptides, and Enzymes

The measurement of pancreatic-derived enzymes and genetic biomarkers in the setting of inflammation form the basis of the laboratory diagnosis of various pancreatic disorders.

- Lipase
- Trypsin
- Stools for fecal fat
- Fecal elastase
- Ingested particles

ICD-9 CODE: Acute Pancreatitis 577.0

ICD-9 CODE: Chronic Pancreatitis 577.1

ICD-9 CODE: Pancreatic Exocrine Disease 577.8

ICD-9 CODE: Steatorrhea 579.4

ICD-9 CODE: Complications of Surgical Procedures/Treatment 998.9

ICD-9 CODE: Complications of Therapeutic Misadventure NEC 999.9

(See Provocative Pancreatic Exocrine Function Tests (Chapter 5) for specific tests and CPT codes)

ADENOCARCINOMA OF THE PANCREAS

Late presentation of pancreatic cancer and its poor prognosis emphasizes the importance of an effective early detection strategy for patients at risk for developing the disease. The recent discovery of genetic biomarkers expressed at different stages of disease was a major advance **(Fig. 2-2).** It is hoped that the clinical uses of genetic and epigenetic biomarkers in combination with the development of high-throughput, sensitive techniques such as proteomics will lead to the rapid discovery of a panel of biomarkers for early detection.

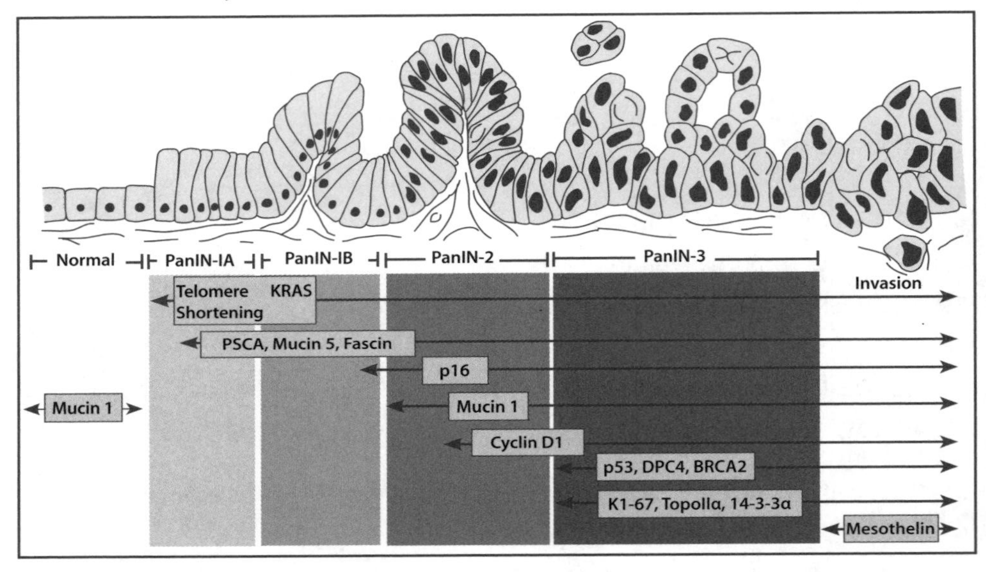

Figure 2-2. Pancreatic Cancer Stages and Overexpressed Genetic Biomarkers (PanIN, pancreatic intraepithelial neoplasia; Adapted from Takaori K, Hruban RH, Maitra A. Pancreatic intraepithelial neoplasia. Pancreas. April;28(3):257-62, 2004.)

WHAT TO LOOK FOR

Distinguishing Signs and Symptoms

- Unexplained weight loss
- Sudden appearance of jaundice
- Abdominal pain

Clinically useful biomarkers and peptides in pancreatic juice and blood include the following:

- KRAS mutations
- P53 mutations
- BRCA2
- Cancer-associated antigen (CA)19-9
- CA-50
- CA-125
- Carcinoembryonic antigen (CEA)

ICD-9 CODE: Adenocarcinoma of the Pancreas 157.4

(See Adenocarcinoma of the Pancreas [Chapter 4] for specific tests and CPT codes)

Pituitary and Hypothalamic Disorders

Diseases of the hypothalamus and pituitary and ectopic production of hypothalamic hormones produce syndromes of hormone excess or deficiency. Nonsecreting pituitary tumors may present with only signs and symptoms of mass effect on adjacent structures (i.e., optic chiasm, cranial nerves 3 and 4 and branches thereof, cranial nerves 5 and 6 as they traverse the cavernous sinus, and the sphenoid sinus) if enough normal pituitary remains to prevent hypopituitarism.

Diseases of Hormonal Excess

- Hyperprolactinemia
- Acromegaly and gigantism
- Cushing's syndrome
- Other pituitary hypersecretion syndromes
  - TSHomas
  - Gonadotropin- or human glycoprotein alpha subunit– (α-GSU) secreting pituitary adenomas

HYPERPROLACTINEMIA

The clinical effects of prolactin excess vary according to the time of onset of the disease.

WHAT TO LOOK FOR

Distinguishing Signs and Symptoms

Children

- Hypogonadism with pubertal delay or arrest
- Absent pubertal growth spurt due to hypogonadism

Women

- Hypogonadism
  - Infertility
  - Oligorrhea/amenorrhea
- Galactorrhea
- Hirsutism due to stimulation of adrenal androgen

ICD-9 CODE: Hyperprolactinemia 253.1

ICD-9 CODE: Hypogonadism
Ovarian 256.1
Testicular 257.2

ICD-9 CODE: Amenorrhea 626.0
Ovarian dysfunction 256.8
Hyperhormonal 256.8

ICD-9 CODE: Oligomenorrhea 626.1

ICD-9 CODE: Galactorrhea 676.6

ICD-9 CODE: Hirsutism 704.1

ICD-9 CODE: MEN-I Syndrome 258.0

(See MEN Syndrome Screen [Chapter 4] and Pituitary and Hypothalamic Disorders Tests [Chapter 5] for specific tests and CPT codes)

ACROMEGALY AND GIGANTISM

Growth hormone is secreted by the anterior pituitary. Its release is controlled by GHRH and somatostatin. GH is also known as somatotropin and is in the family of compounds known as somatomammotropins, which includes prolactin and human placental lactogen. GH stimulates production of RNA, resulting in increased anabolism. GH levels are elevated in persons with pituitary gigantism and in those with acromegaly that is characterized by growth after the epiphyses have closed resulting in abnormal bone growth of face, hands, and feet. GH levels are decreased in persons with dwarfism. Patients taking GH therapy frequently develop GH antibodies, which act to negate the biologic effect of the medication.

The clinical effects of GH excess vary according to the time of onset of the disease. Relative frequency of symptoms in acromegaly is shown in **Table 2-4**.

Table 2-4. The Relative Frequency of Symptoms in Acromegaly

Clinical Features	Percentage
Enlargement of extremities	99
Facial coarsening	97
Visceromegaly	92
Necessity to increase shoe size	88
Necessity to increase ring size	87
Sella enlargement	83
Acroparesthesias	82
Arthralgia	80
Hyperhidrosis, seborrhea	78
Arthrosis	76
Teeth separation	75
Frontal bossing	72
Oily skin	70
Malocclusion and overbite	65
Prognathism	65
Headache	62
Sleep apnea	52
High blood pressure	42
Impaired glucose tolerance	40
Skin tags	38
Goiter	38
Menstrual abnormalities	36
Asthenia	35
Sexual disturbances	34
Carpal tunnel syndrome	28
Overt diabetes	28
Visual field defects	27
Galactorrhea	4
Cranial nerve palsies	3

WHAT TO LOOK FOR

Distinguishing Signs and Symptoms

The somatic changes in children include the following:

- Increase in growth velocity
- Gigantism

The changes in adults and children include the following:

- Enlargement of the extremities (hands, feet, nose, mandible, and supraorbital ridges) compelling patients to seek large gloves, shoes, and rings
- Development of thick skin which is moist, oily, and seborrheic with an increase in sebaceous cysts and skin tags
- Acanthosis nigricans and hypertrichosis
- Widely spaced teeth
- Visceromegaly of the tongue, liver, thyroid, and salivary glands
- Overgrowth of bone and cartilage causing degenerative changes in spine, hips, and knees
- Arthralgia and paresthesias
- Nerve entrapments, particularly of the median nerve but also ulnar and peroneal

Diagnosis of Acromegaly

The basal level of GH and IGF-1 is usually sufficient to make the diagnosis. However, in 15% to 25% of cases, the levels of GH are less than 10 ng/mL and the IGF-1 level may be normal. In these instances it is important to show nonsuppressibility of GH to an oral glucose tolerance test (or a somatostatin inhibition or bromocryptine suppression test). Levels of other pituitary hormones such as prolactin and the α subunit of gonadotropins are also often elevated; measure these as well as thyroid-stimulating hormone (TSH). If ordering a glucose tolerance test, measure GH in addition to glucose, because the criterion for diagnosis of acromegaly is based on suppression of GH and insulin as well as lipids.

THE NEXT STEP

Imaging of the sella turcica will show a tumor. In the absence of a tumor and the suggestion of hyperplasia, evaluate for a hypothalamic hamartoma or ectopic production of GHRH. If the GHRH level is greater than 300 pg/mL, CT and MRI of the pancreas, gastroduodenal area, thymus, and lungs should facilitate a diagnosis. Because these NETs express somatostatin receptors, OctreoScan will often reveal their location. In about 20% of patients a pituitary tumor will coexist with MEN-I syndrome; thus it is important to also measure ionized calcium and PTH.

The radiologic study of bones will show thickening of the skull, enlargement of the frontal and maxillary sinuses, prognathism, tufting of the phalanges, and cysts in carpal and tarsal bones. Soft tissue enlargement can be seen, particularly with heel pad thickness. In patients over 50 years old, colonic polyps may become carcinomas, particularly in people with skin tags. For these patients, routine sequential colonoscopy is recommended. The flow diagram presented in **Figure 2-3** suggests the diagnostic workup.

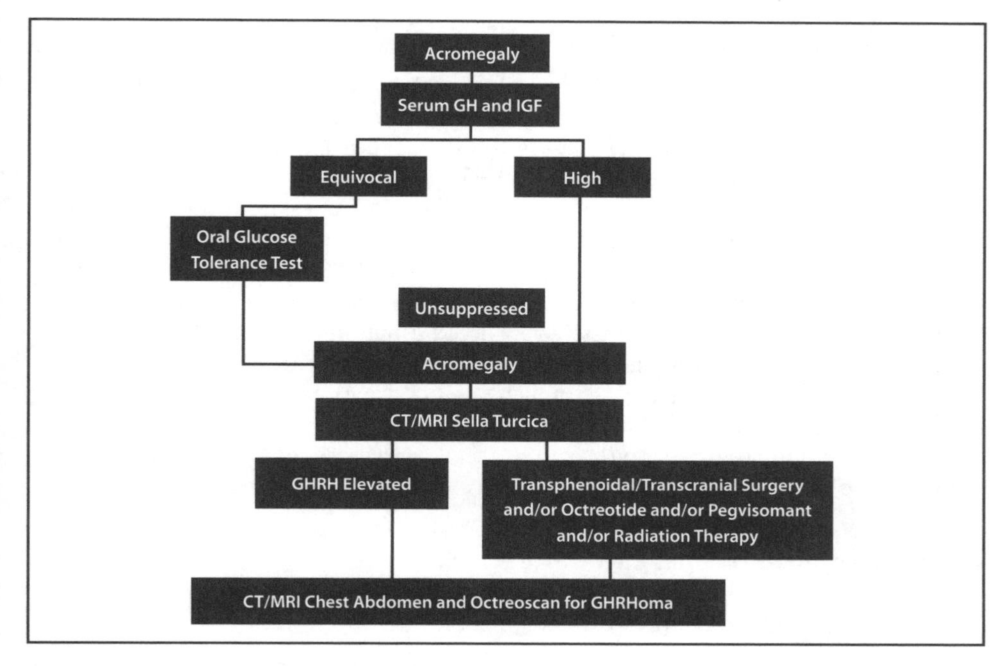

Figure 2-3. Flow Diagram for Diagnostic Workup

Hormones and Peptides

- GH
- IGF-1
- Prolactin
- TSH
- GHRH if no tumor visualized or pituitary hyperplasia on MRI
- PTH

Measure the following:

- GH and IGF-1
- Oral glucose tolerance test; also measure GH, insulin, and lipids
- Somatostatin inhibition test
- Bromocryptine suppression test
- Prolactin
- TSH
- Ionized calcium
- PTH

ICD-9 CODE: Acromegaly 253.0

ICD-9 CODE: Gigantism 253.0

ICD-9 CODE: MEN-I Syndrome 258.0

(See Growth Hormone [HGH, Somatotropin] [Chapter 3] and Thyroid Stimulating Hormone [TSH, Thyrotropin] [Chapter 3] for specific tests and CPT codes)

CUSHING'S SYNDROME

In Cushing's disease, oversecretion of pituitary ACTH induces bilateral adrenal hyperplasia. This results in excess production of cortisol, adrenal androgens, and 11-deoxycorticosterone. Cushing's disease, a subset of Cushing's syndrome, is due to a pituitary corticotroph adenoma and results in a partial resistance to the suppression of ACTH by cortisol so that secretion is unrestrained. In contrast, causes of Cushing's syndrome may include the following:

- Adrenal adenoma or carcinoma arise spontaneously. ACTH levels are undetectable.
- Nonpituitary (ectopic) tumors produce ACTH. They most frequently originate in the thorax and are highly aggressive small cell carcinomas of the lung or slow-growing bronchial or thymic carcinoid tumors. Some produce corticotropin-releasing hormone (CRH) instead, which stimulates pituitary ACTH secretion and can therefore mimic a pituitary tumor.
- Other causes include carcinoid tumors of the gastric, pancreatic, and intestinal organs; pheochromocytomas; and MCT.

The hallmark of Cushing's syndrome is that ACTH levels are partially resistant to suppression with dexamethasone, even at very high doses.

WHAT TO LOOK FOR

Distinguishing Signs and Symptoms

The clinical features of common varieties of Cushing's disease include or are related to the following:

- Fat and protein metabolism
- Centripetal weight gain
- Development of the buffalo hump
- Supraclavicular fat pads
- Plethoric moon face
- Thin skin
- Little accumulation of subcutaneous fat over the dorsum of the hand and shin
- Purple striae, often greater than 1 cm wide, usually located over the abdomen but not in traditional stretch areas
- Slow healing of minor wounds
- Muscle wasting in the proximal lower limbs leading to inability to rise from a chair and weakness
- Bone wasting resulting in generalized osteoporosis
- Kyphosis and loss of height
- Elevated blood pressure
- Fluid accumulation leading to congestive heart failure
- Evidence of androgen excess with hirsutism in women
- Clitoromegaly
- Coarsening of the skin
- Hoarse voice douse to the androgen excess, particularly true in adrenocortical carcinomas
- Psychic disturbances

- Anxiety
- Emotional lability
- Depression
- Unwarranted euphoria with sleep disturbances

The nonpituitary or ectopic ACTH syndrome is often diagnosed because of its rapid onset and progress. Classically the condition is dominated by the following characteristics:

- Profound muscle wasting
- Electrolyte disturbances
- Severe hypokalemia
- Overproduction of mineralocorticoids
- Impaired insulin secretion resulting in diabetes
- Striking pigmentation due to the structural homology of ACTH and MSH

This pigmentation contrasts with the absence of pigmentation in classic Cushing's disease and adrenal tumors, in which ACTH is suppressed.

The Next Step

Increased urinary cortisol and plasma cortisol suggest Cushing's disease. A suppressed ACTH level indicates the presence of an adrenal tumor. Mildly elevated ACTH directs attention to the pituitary. Markedly elevated ACTH suggests a small cell carcinoma of the lung or an ectopic carcinoid type of tumor.

Hormones and Peptides

- ACTH
- Cortisol
- Adrenal
- Androgens
- 11-Deoxycorticosterone
- MSH

First-Line Screening

1. Measure plasma ACTH, cortisol, and 24-hour urinary free cortisol excretion.
2. Repeat at least three 24-hour urinary free cortisol collections if high clinical suspicion exists. One or more collections may be normal due to "cyclic Cushing's disease," and in preclinical Cushing's syndrome, the urinary free cortisol may be normal.
3. Perform low-dose dexamethasone suppression test (DST) either overnight (1 mg between 11:00 PM and 12:00 AM) or 0.5 mg every 6 hours for 48 hours. N–1 suppression is to less than 1.8 µg/dL (50 nmol/L).
4. Measure circadian rhythm of cortisol by obtaining serum cortisols at 8:00 to 9:30 AM, 4:30 to 6:00 PM, and 11:00 PM to 12:00 AM. For the latter measurement, patient should be asleep as an inpatient after 48 hours (only if not acutely ill); if patient is not in the hospital, or is acutely ill, obtain a salivary cortisol level.

(See Pituitary and Hypothalamic Tests [Chapter 5] for more details on ACTH and cortisol testing)

Second-Line Screening

1. Measure circadian rhythm of cortisol, as above.
2. Perform low-dose DST 0.5 mg for 48 hours with measurement of 24-hour urinary free cortisol on the second day. Excretion of less than 10 μg/24 hours (27 nmol/L) is normal.
3. Perform low-dose DST (0.5 mg every 6 hours for 48 hours) followed by CRH stimulation (100 μg or 1 μg/kg of intravenous ovine CRH). A cortisol response greater than 1.4 μg/dL at 15 minutes is consistent with Cushing's disease.

(See Pituitary and Hypothalamic Tests [Chapter 5] for more details on cortisol testing, low-dose DST, and low-dose DST with CRH stimulation)

What You Need to Know if Cushing's Syndrome Is Confirmed

1. If ACTH is easily detectable (>20 pg/mL, or 4 pmol/L) focus on the pituitary with MRI of the sella turcica. This test is positive in 50% to 60% of cases of proven pituitary Cushing's disease.
2. If ACTH level is less than 20 pg/mL, prove that it is suppressed with a CRH test. Administer CRH 1 μg/kg or 100 μg/1 kg (but *not* dexamethasone) as described previously, and measure ACTH in addition to cortisol at 15, 30, and 45 minutes after CRH. An increase of greater than 50% in ACTH supports a pituitary tumor; ectopic ACTH-secreting tumors generally (but not invariably) do not respond to CRH. Those that do are carcinoids tumors of bronchus, thymus, or pancreas; islet cell tumors; MCTs; or pheochromocytomas rather than the more common small cell carcinomas of the lung.
3. Perform high-dose DST. High doses of glucocorticoids partially suppress ACTH secretion from 80% to 90% of corticotroph adenomas, whereas ectopic tumors usually resist negative feedback inhibition. However, as discussed previously, some benign NETs may be sensitive to feedback inhibition of ACTH, similar to pituitary tumors. In adrenal-based Cushing's syndrome, plasma cortisol is not suppressed after high-dose DST because cortisol secretion is autonomous and pituitary ACTH secretion is already suppressed. As with the low-dose DST, there are several versions of the high-dose DST, including the standard 2-day oral high dose (2 mg every 6 hours for 48 hours), the 8-mg overnight oral, the intravenous 4 mg, and the ultra-high-dose (8 mg every 6 hours) tests. Plasma and/or urinary cortisol levels are evaluated before, during, and/or after DST. Suppression of plasma cortisol to 50% of baseline provides a specificity of up to 80%.
4. Perform inferior petrosal sinus sampling. If the above tests point to an ACTH-dependent process but no adenoma is evident on MRI, the next step should be bilateral inferior petrosal sinus sampling. An experienced radiologist catheterizes both inferior petrosal sinuses, and samples for ACTH are obtained simultaneously from both the sinuses and a peripheral vein before and at 3, 5, and 10 minutes after intravenous administration of ovine CRH (1 μg/kg or 100 μg/1 kg). An inferior petrosal sinus–to–peripheral ACTH ratio greater than 2.0 at baseline or after CRH administration is consistent with Cushing's disease. Lower ratios suggest an ectopic ACTH-secreting tumor. A side-to-side ratio of 1.4 or greater may provide direction to neurosurgeons performing transsphenoidal hypophysectomy when no tumor is evident on MRI.

In Search of Occult Ectopic ACTH-Secreting Tumors

If bilateral inferior petrosal sinus sampling confirms the lack of a pituitary ACTH gradient, perform CT and/or MRI of the neck, thorax, and abdomen, because most nonpituitary ACTH-secreting tumors are NETs, as noted previously. Additionally, perform MRI of the chest, because this imaging procedure may uncover (central) bronchial carcinoids missed by CT. Somatostatin analog scintigraphy with ^{111}In-pentetreotide (OctreoScan) may identify a few occult ACTH-secreting tumors with somatostatin receptors that were not clearly identified by CT or MRI imaging. Positron emission tomography scanning may also prove helpful in the search for occult ACTH-secreting tumors.

Other procedures that have been used to discriminate between pituitary-dependent and ectopic ACTH syndromes include desmopressin with or without CRH; the GH secretatogogues hexarelin and ghrelin, which stimulate ACTH in patients with pituitary adenomas but not in normals; and the opiate agonist loperamide, which suppresses normals but not patients with Cushing's disease. None of these research procedures can be recommended for standard clinical practice as of yet.

ICD-9 CODE: Cushing's Syndrome/Cushing's Disease 255.0

(See Pituitary and Hypothalamic Disorders Tests [Chapter 5] for specific tests and CPT codes)

Other Pituitary Hypersecretion Syndromes

TSH-Secreting Pituitary Adenomas (TSHoma)

Thyroid-stimulating hormone is a glycoprotein produced in the pituitary consisting of two subunits: α and β. The α subunit is identical or similar to that of follicle-stimulating hormone (FSH), luteinizing hormone (LH), and chorionic gonadotropin. The β subunit is specific to TSH. The secretion of TSH is controlled by release of thyrotropin-releasing hormone (TRH) from the hypothalamus. TSH stimulates all metabolic and cellular processes involved in synthesis and secretion of thyroid hormones. TSH also stimulates intermediary metabolism and thyroid growth. TSH initiates release of thyroxine and triiodothyronine from thyroglobulin. TSH is increased in almost all cases of primary hypothyroidism and decreased in most cases of hyperthyroidism; TSH thyrotoxicosis is one exception. TSH secretion is increased by estrogens and suppressed by androgens and corticosteroids.

Thyrotropin-releasing hormone is a tripeptide produced primarily by the hypothalamus. TRH is produced from a prohormone that contains multiple copies of the TRH molecule. Several TRH entities can be released from one precursor. TRH has a stimulatory effect on the pituitary, causing it to release TSH. TRH secretion is controlled by hormones via a negative feedback system. Binding of TRH to its receptor causes a rise in calcium, which initiates TSH secretion. It also stimulates adenyl cyclase in the pituitary. Additionally, TRH stimulates secretion of prolactin, GH in acromegaly, and ACTH in Cushing's and Nelson's syndromes. Levels of TRH are undetectable or very low in patients with hyperthyroidism and hypothalamic hypothyroidism. Levels are elevated in patients with primary and pituitary hypothyroidism.

What to Look For

Distinguishing Signs and Symptoms

- Approximately 300 cases have been reported in the last 35 years. Previously, TSHomas were not found until they had grown to macroadenoma size (>10 mm); more recently, some of these tumors are discovered at the microadenoma size as a result of the 100-fold increase in sensitivity in TSH assays.
- When pituitary adenomas secrete TSH, they are autonomous and refractory to the negative feedback of thyroid hormones (i.e., inappropriate TSH secretion) and can produce hyperthyroidism. Thus, the key finding is detectable serum TSH levels in the presence of elevated free tri-iodothyronine (T4) and free thyroixine (T3) concentrations. TSH concentrations may be elevated or normal.
- Earlier diagnosis and treatment directed at the pituitary, as opposed to the thyroid, may prevent the loss of visual field caused by impingement on the optic chiasm and hypopituitarism that occur as the tumors enlarge, and furthermore may improve the rate of neurosurgical cure.

- TSHomas present with signs and symptoms of hyperthyroidism including goiter, and 25% of these tumors show mixed pituitary hormone secretion, usually GH or prolactin, thus patients should be evaluated for galactorrhea/amenorrhea and acromegaly.

The Next Step

Hormones and Peptides

- TSH
- Free T4 and free T3
- Prolactin
- GH and IGF-1
- α-GSU
- LH, FSH
- Testosterone, sex hormone–binding globulin, or estradiol
- Cortisol and ACTH

Dynamic testing may be required to uncover hypocortisolism. See Pituitary and Hypothalamic Disorders, discussed earlier in this chapter.

Dynamic Testing

- T3 suppression test (75–100 μg/d orally in divided doses for 8–10 days). Inhibition of TSH secretion after T3 suppression test has never been recorded in patients with TSHoma. However, this test is strictly contraindicated in elderly patients or in those with coronary heart disease.
- TRH test. Widely used to investigate the presence of a TSHoma. The TRH collection instructions are available on page 163. After intravenous administration of 200 μg TRH, TSH and α-GSU levels generally do not increase in patients with TSHoma.
- Somatostatin suppression test. Administration of somatostatin or its analogs (octreotide and lanreotide) reduces TSH levels in most cases and may predict the efficacy of long-term treatment, but it is not considered diagnostic for TSHoma.

Imaging Studies and Localization of the Tumor

Nuclear MRI is preferred for imaging other tumors of the sella turcica, such as TSHomas. CT may be used as an alternative to MRI in patients with a contraindication (e.g., pacemaker, claustrophobia).

For more information go to:
http://www.thyroidmanager.org/Chapter13/13A-text.htm

Gonadotropin or α-GSU–Secreting Pituitary Adenomas

Many pituitary adenomas stain positively for either LH or FSH or for their α-glycoprotein subunit (and also that of TSH and human chorionic gonadotropin) few patients have elevated gonadotropin levels. Gonadotropinomas (or α-GSUomas) generally present as macroadenomas with visual field loss, headaches, or hypopituitarism including infertility, early menopause, or male hypogonadism. In general, elevations of both LH and FSH imply primary hypogonadism rather than gonadotropinoma. Because α-GSU is frequently secreted in mixed or "silent" pituitary adenomas, its concentration should be measured as part of the evaluation of any pituitary adenoma.

ICD-9 CODE: Pituitary Syndrome 253.0

ICD-9 CODE: Other/Unspecified Anterior Pituitary Hyperfunction 253.1

ICD-9 CODE: Thyrotoxicosis of Other Specified Origin Without Mention of Crisis or Storm; Overproduction of TSH 242.80

ICD-9 CODE: Thyrotoxicosis of Other Specified Origin Without Mention of Crisis or Storm; Overproduction of TSH 242.81
ICD-9 CODES for Pituitary Neoplasm

Site	Malignant	Benign	Uncertain Behavior	Unspecified
Pituitary gland	194.3	227.3	237.0	239.74

(See Pituitary and Hypothalamic Disorders Tests [Chapter 5] for specific tests and CPT codes)

PITUITARY HORMONE INSUFFICIENCY (CHILDHOOD)

Multiple childhood tumors can affect pituitary function, including craniopharyngioma, germinoma, hamartoma, low-grade astrocytoma, Langerhans' cell histiocytosis, and dermoid and epidermoid tumors. These generally compress the hypothalamus or, in the case of craniopharyngioma and germinoma, the pituitary stalk. Benign pituitary adenomas frequently affect the anterior pituitary. Common posterior pituitary lesions include astrocytoma and Langerhans' cell histiocytosis.

WHAT TO LOOK FOR

Distinguishing Signs and Symptoms

- Raised intracranial pressure caused by expansion of tumor with obstruction of the cerebrospinal fluid (CSF), causing headaches, vomiting, and papilledema.
- Cranial nerve palsies, visual field defects, and hypothalamo-hypophyseal dysfunction (one third of cases as the initial presentation).
- Hyposecretion (and occasionally hypersecretion) of pituitary hormones. These are usually easy to recognize.
- Hypothalamo-pituitary syndromes, characterized by variable endocrine disturbances, occur in association with hypothalamic dysfunction. (The hypothalamus is important for the control of many basic cerebral functions, such as appetite, emotion, and temperature homoeostasis).
- Craniopharyngioma and peripituitary lesions with suprasellar extension may cause visual difficulties due to the compression of the optic nerves and/or chiasm.
- Hypopituitarism. Usually, hormone loss is sequential, beginning with loss of GH secretion, followed by gonadotropins, TSH, and ACTH. In children, in contrast to adults, the loss of GH secretion is usually more obvious with growth failure and possibly hypoglycemia.
- Central precocious puberty, defined as signs of puberty (breast development in girls, and increase in testicular volume in boys) occurring under the age of 8 years in a girl and 8.5 years in a boy. These symptoms are gonadotropin dependent and therefore are ameliorated by long-acting gonadotropin-releasing hormone agonists, which downregulate the pituitary gonadotropin-releasing hormone receptors.
- Hypothalamopituitary tumors in the peripubertal age range may present as failure to enter puberty or arrested pubertal development and consequent blunted or even absent growth spurt.

If onset of gonadotropin-releasing hormone insufficiency occurs during fetal development (i.e., congenital), the male genitalia will be abnormal, with micropenis and bilateral small undescended testes due to failure of testosterone secretion in utero. Under these circumstances, perform MRI of the olfactory bulbs/grooves to seek evidence of Kallmann's syndrome.

ICD-9 CODE: Hypopituitarism 253.2
Hormone therapy 253.7
Hypophysectomy 253.7
Radiotherapy 253.7
Postablative 253.7
Postpartum hemorrhage 253.2

(See Pituitary and Hypothalamic Disorders Tests [Chapter 5] for specific tests (mentioned above) and CPT codes)

DIABETES INSIPIDUS (ADULTHOOD)

Vasopressin is derived from the supraoptic and periventricular nuclei of the hypothalamus and is released from the nerve endings in the neurohypophysis (i.e., posterior pituitary). Before overt diabetes insipidus occurs, 85% to 90% of vasopressin secretion must be lost. New-onset diabetes insipidus should raise suspicion of a tumor, although 50% of acquired cases have an autoimmune etiology. Tumors may be occult for many years; thus, patients often require serial neuroimaging to reveal the diagnosis.

CAUSES

Hypothalamic (Central) Diabetes Insipidus (HDI)

- Congenital
  - Genetic: Wolfram syndrome or diabetes insipidus, diabetes mellitus, optic atrophy, and deafness (DIDMOAD)
  - Developmental syndromes: septo-optic dysplasia, Lawrence-Moon-Biedel syndrome
- Idiopathic
- Acquired
  - Trauma
  - Neurosurgical injury (transcranial, transsphenoidal)
- Tumor
  - Craniopharyngioma, pinealoma, germinoma, metastases, pituitary macroadenoma (unusual cause as it is a hypothalamic disease)
- Inflammatory
  - Granulomas
  - Sarcoid
  - Tuberculous meningitis
  - Langerhans' cell histiocytosis
  - Meningitis, encephalitis
- Infundibuloneurohypophysitis
- Autoimmune
  - Anti-vasopressin neuron antibodies
- Vascular
  - Aneurysm
  - Infarction: Sheehan's syndrome, sickle cell disease
- Pregnancy (associated with vasopressinase)

Nephrogenic Diabetes Insipidus (NDI)

- Genetic
  - X-linked recessive (V2-R defect)
  - Autosomal recessive (AQP2 defect)
  - Autosomal dominant (AQP2 defect)
- Idiopathic
- Chronic renal disease (e.g., polycystic kidneys)

- Metabolic disease
  - Hypercalcemia
  - Hypokalemia
- Drug induced
  - Lithium
  - Demeclocycline
  - Platinum-based antineoplastic drugs
- Osmotic diuretics
  - Glucose
  - Mannitol
  - Urea (post–obstructive uropathy)
- Systemic disorders
  - Amyloidosis
  - Myelomatosis
- Pregnancy

Dipsogenic Diabetes Insipidus (DDI)

- Compulsive water drinking associated with psychologic disorders (i.e., psychogenic polydypsia)
- Drug induced

Structural/Organic Hypothalamic Disease

- Tumors involving hypothalamus
- Head injury

Granulomatous Diseases

- Sarcoid
- Tuberculous meningitis
- Langerhans' cell histiocytosis

WHAT TO LOOK FOR

Distinguishing Signs and Symptoms

- Thirst
- Polydipsia
- Polyuria

Exclude the following conditions:

- Hyperglycemia
- Hypokalemia
- Hypercalcemia
- Renal insufficiency

Measure the following values:

- 24-Hour urine volume (abnormal is >40 mL/kg/24 hours)
- Serum sodium (generally maintained in the high-normal range in HDI, but generally maintained in the low-normal range in DDI)

- Glucose
- Blood urea nitrogen (BUN)
- Serum and urine osmolality
- Plasma vasopressin

The Next Step

Request water deprivation/desmopressin test to determine whether HDI, NDI, or DDI.

- HDI: urine osmolality is less than 300 mOsm/kg accompanied by plasma osmolality greater than 290 mOsm/kg after dehydration; urine osmolality should rise above 750 mOsm/kg after desmopressin acetate (DDAVP)
- NDI: failure to increase urine osmolality above 300 mOsm/kg after dehydration, with no response to DDAVP
- DDI: appropriate urine concentration during dehydration without significant rise in plasma osmolality

If HDI is diagnosed, the next step should be imaging of the hypothalamus/perisellar region with MRI to exclude possible tumors. HDI frequently is associated with loss of the normal posterior pituitary bright spot on T1-weighted MRI, which correlates with posterior pituitary vasopressin content.

For more information go to:
http://www.endotext.com/neuroendo/neuroendo11a/neuroendoframe11a.htm (Children)
http://www.endotext.com/neuroendo/neuroendo2/neuroendoframe2.htm (Diabetes Insipidus and Syndrome of Inappropriate Antidiuretic Hormone [SIADH])

ICD-9 CODE: Diabetes Insipidus 253.5

ICD-9 CODE: Nephrogenic Diabetes Insipidus 588.1

ICD-9 CODE: Pituitary Diabetes Insipidus 253.5

ICD-9 CODE Vasopressin-Resistant Diabetes Insipidus 588.1

(See Water Deprivation/Desmopression Test for Diabetes Insipidus: Hypothalamic [HDI], Nephrogenic [NDI], and Dipsogenic [DDI] [Chapter 5] for specific tests and CPT codes)

HYPONATREMIA AND SYNDROME OF INAPPROPRIATE ANTIDIURETIC HORMONE

Hyponatremia (serum sodium level <135 mEq/L) and hypo-osmolality are the most common fluid and electrolyte disorders in hospitalized patients with hyponatremia and syndrome of inappropriate antidiuretic hormone (SIADH). Hyponatremia is important clinically because severe hypo-osmolality (serum sodium level <120 mEq/L) is associated with substantial morbidity and mortality. Excessively rapid correction of hyponatremia can itself cause severe neurologic morbidity and mortality due to osmotic demyelinization (i.e., central pontine demyelinization).

WHAT TO LOOK FOR

Distinguishing Signs and Symptoms

- Lethargy
- Anorexia
- Headache
- Nausea
- Vomiting
- Muscle cramps
- Disorientation
- Seizure
- Coma
- Death

Criteria for Diagnosis of Hyponatremia Due to SIADH

- Hyponatremia with appropriately low plasma osmolality (<280 mOsm/kg)
- Urine osmolality greater than 100 mOsm/kg (i.e., less than maximally dilute) at a time when the plasma is hypo-osmolar
- Renal (urine) sodium excretion greater than 30 mM/L
- Absence of hypotension, hypovolemia, and edema-forming states
- Normal cardiac, renal, pituitary, thyroid, and adrenal function

Differential Diagnosis

Plasma osmolality can be calculated as (mOsm/kg H_3O) = 2x $[Na^+]$ (mEq/L) + glucose (mg/dL)/18 + BUN (mg/dL)/2.8 and is accurate under usual conditions but can be misleading under the following conditions:

- Pseudohyponatremia, which is due to gross hyperlipidemia (triglycerides or cholesterol) or serum proteins
- Isotonic or hypertonic hyponatremia, which is due to high concentrations of other solutes (e.g., glucose, mannitol, alcohols/ethylene glycol, radiocontrast dyes, urea)

Hypotonic hyponatremia is best determined by directly measuring plasma osmolality. If direct and calculated measurements agree, then calculated osmolality can be used subsequently.

Measure the following levels:

- Plasma osmolality
- Serum sodium
- Glucose
- BUN
- Ethanol, methanol, etc. (depending on the situation)
- Urine osmolality
- Urine sodium
- Serum uric acid

Causes of Hypotonic Hyponatremia

- Sodium depletion
  - Renal loss
  - Diuretics
  - Salt-wasting nephropathy
  - Central salt wasting
- Extrarenal loss
  - GI losses (vomiting, diarrhea)
  - Sweating
  - Hemorrhage
- Hypoadrenalism (renal losses if primary, decreased free water excretion in primary or secondary)
- Reduced renal free water clearance
  - Hypovolemia
  - Cardiac failure
  - Nephrotic syndrome
  - Hypothyroidism
  - Renal failure
  - Ascites
  - Hypoalbuminemia
  - Sepsis and vascular leak syndromes
  - Fluid sequestration
- Excess water intake
  - DDI at times when water intake exceeds renal clearance
  - Sodium-free, hyposomolar irrigant solutions
  - Dilute infant feeding formula
  - SIADH

Causes of Drug-Induced Hyponatremia

- Saline depletion: diuretics, spironolactone, thiazides, loop diuretics plus angiotensin-converting enzyme (ACE) inhibitors, angiotensin receptor blockers

Causes of Vasopressin-Like Activity

- DDAVP
- Oxytocin
- Potentiation of vasopressin action
- Nonsteroidal anti-inflammatory agents
- Carbamazepine
- Chlorpropamide
- Cyclophosphamide
- Ifosfamide
- Cisplatin
- Carboplatin
- Vincristine
- Vinblastine

Causes of SIADH Other Than Drugs

- Neoplastic disease
- Chest disorders
    - Carcinoma (bronchus, duodenum, pancreas, bladder, ureter, prostate)
    - Thymoma
    - Mesothelioma
    - Lymphoma, leukemia
    - Carcinoid
    - Bronchial adenoma
    - Pneumonia
    - Tuberculosis
    - Empyema
    - Cystic fibrosis
    - Pneumothorax
- Neurological disorders
    - Head injury, neurosurgery
    - Brain abscess or tumor
    - Meningitis, encephalitis
    - Guillain-Barré syndrome
    - Cerebral hemorrhage
    - Cavernous sinus thrombosis
    - Hydrocephalus
    - Cerebellar and cerebral atrophy
    - Shy-Drager syndrome
    - Peripheral neuropathy
    - Seizures
    - Subdural hematoma
    - Alcohol withdrawal

- Miscellaneous
    - Idiopathic
    - Psychosis
    - Porphyria
    - Abdominal surgery
- Drug-induced
    - Dopamine antagonists: phenothiazines, butyrophenones, etc.
    - Antidepressants: tricyclics, monoamineoxidase inhibitors, selective serotonin reuptake inhibitors, venlafaxine
    - Opiates
    - Antiepileptics: carbamazepine, oxcarbazipine, sodium valproate
    - 3,4-Methylenedioxymethamphetamine (MDMA; ecstasy)
    - Clofibrate
    - Cyclophosphamide
    - Chlorpropamide

Table 2-5 provides a diagnostic schema for hyponatremia.

Table 2-5. Diagnostic Schema for Hyponatremia

		Hypovolemia		Euvolemia		Hypervolemia	
Extracellular Na+		↓↓		→		↑	
Total body water		↓		↑		↑↑	
Common causes	• Renal loss • Diuretics • Mineralocorticoid deficiency • Salt-losing nephritis • Cerebral salt wasting		• Extra-renal loss • Vomiting • Diarrhea • Burns	• SIADH • Hypothyroidism • Glucocorticoid deficiency • Sick cell syndrome	• Cardiac failure • Cirrhosis • Nephrotic syndrome		• Renal failure
Urinary Na+ (mmol/L)	>20		<10	>20	<10		>20
Plasma osmolarity (mOsm/kg)	>280		>280	>280	<280		
Urine osmolarity (mOsm/kg)	>280		<280	>280	<280		

ICD-9 CODE: Hyponatremia 271.1

ICD-9 CODE: SIADH 253.6

(See test sections mentioned above and Waterload Test for Impaired Water Clearance [Chapter 5] for specific tests and CPT codes)

Obesity

In the United States, approximately two of three persons over the age of 40 years are overweight. Furthermore, there is increasing concern about the number of children and adolescents with excess adiposity. Obesity it is associated with high costs in morbidity, including a significantly increased risk of type 2 diabetes and cardiovascular disease. The comorbidities of diabetes and their prevalences are provided in **Table 2-6** and **Figure 2-4**.

Table 2-6. Comorbidities of Diabetes

- Cardiovascular
  - Hypertension
  - Congestive heart failure
  - Cor pulmonale
  - Varicose veins
  - Pulmonary embolism
  - Coronary artery disease
- Neurologic
  - Stroke
  - Idiopathic intracranial hypertension
  - Meralgia paresthetica
- Musculoskeletal
  - Hyperuricemia and gout
  - Immobility
  - Degenerative arthritis
  - Low back pain
- Integumentary
  - Stasis pigmentation of legs
  - Cellulitis
  - Acanthosis nigricans/skin tags
  - Intertrigo, carbuncles
  - Striae distensae (stretch marks)
  - Lymphedema
- Psychological
  - Depression/low self-esteem
  - Impaired quality of life
  - Social stigmatization
- Respiratory
  - Dyspnea and fatigue
  - Obstructive sleep apnea
  - Hypoventilation syndrome
  - Pickwickian syndrome
  - Asthma
- Endocrine
  - Metabolic syndrome
  - Type 2 diabetes
  - Dyslipidemia
  - Polycystic ovarian syndrome/hyperandrogenism
  - Amenorrhea/infertility/menstrual disorders
- Gastrointestinal
  - Gastroesophageal reflux disease
  - Nonalcoholic fatty liver disease
  - Cholelithiasis
  - Hernias
  - Colon cancer
- Genitourinary
  - Urinary stress incontinence
  - Hypogonadism (male)
  - Breast and uterine cancer
  - Pregnancy complications
  - Obesity-related glomerulopathy

From Kushner RF, Weinsier RL. Evaluation of the obese patient. Practical considerations. Med Clin North Am. Mar;84(2): 387-99, 2000.

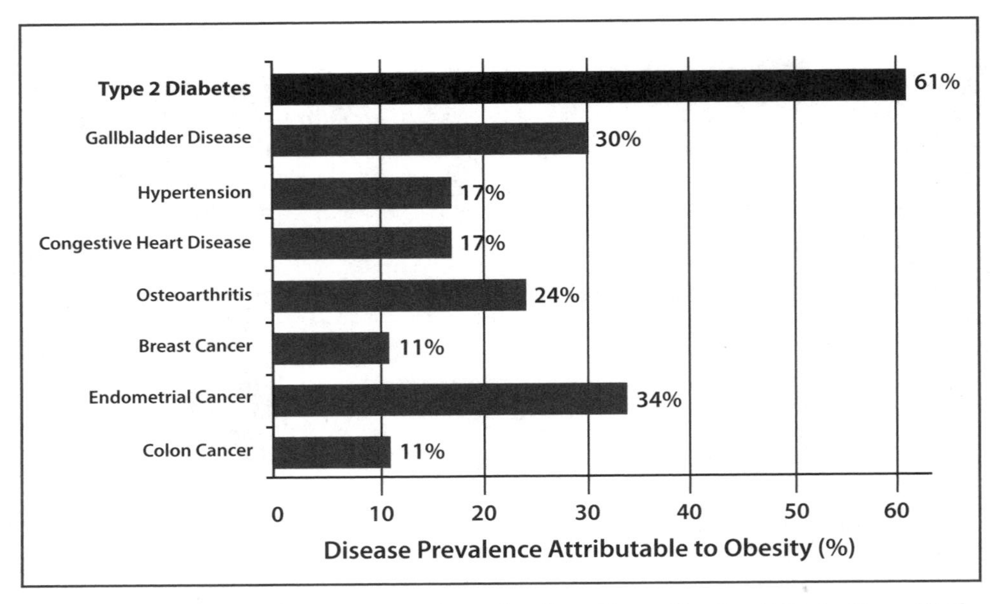

Figure 2-4. Proportion of Disease Prevalence Attributable to Obesity (Adapted from Wolf AM, Colditz GA. Current estimates of the economic cost of obesity in the United States. Obes Res. 6:97-106, 1998.)

How Is Obesity Defined?

Obesity is defined in several different ways. The most common method is calculation of the body mass index (BMI) using the following formula: BMI = ((weight in pounds)/(height in inches) x (height in inches)) x 703. Typically, a table of BMI levels is used. **Figure 2-5** allows persons to determine their degree of overweight.

Height \ Weight (lb)	120	130	140	150	160	170	180	190	200	210	220	230	240	250	260	270	280	290	300
5'0"	23	25	27	29	31	33	35	37	39	41	43	45	47	49	51	53	55	57	59
5'2"	22	24	26	27	29	31	33	35	37	38	40	42	44	46	48	49	51	53	55
5'4"	21	22	24	26	28	29	31	33	34	36	38	40	41	43	45	46	48	50	52
5'6"	19	21	23	24	26	27	29	31	32	34	36	37	39	40	42	44	45	47	49
5'8"	18	20	21	23	24	26	27	29	31	32	34	35	37	38	40	41	43	44	46
5'10"	17	19	20	22	23	24	26	27	29	30	32	33	35	36	37	39	40	42	43
6'0"	16	18	19	20	22	23	24	26	27	29	30	31	33	34	35	37	38	39	41
6'2"	15	17	18	19	21	22	23	24	26	27	28	30	31	32	33	35	36	37	39
6'4"	15	16	17	18	20	21	22	23	24	26	27	28	29	30	32	33	34	35	37

Figure 2-5. Body Mass Index Levels

The National Institutes of Health, specifically the National Heart Lung and Blood Institutes and the National Institute for Diabetes and Digestive and Kidney Diseases, together with the North American Association for the Study of Obesity, released guidelines for the treatment of obesity in 2002. These guidelines identify degrees of obesity using BMI as shown in Figure 2-5. This chart provides an easy way to calculate BMI. The area shaded in dark blue represents patients with a BMI >30. These patients are classified as obese and are at high risk for obesity-associated mortality and comorbid diseases. The area shaded in medium blues or dark gray represents patients with BMIs of 25 to 29.9. These patients are classified as overweight with an increased risk of obesity-associated mortality and comorbid diseases. The area shaded in light gray represents patients with normal BMIs (18.5–24.9). A patient with a BMI in the white area is underweight. As an example, a person who is 6 feet tall and weighs 180 lb has a BMI of 24 (see black circle, **Fig. 2-5**). With increasing abdominal obesity in particular, macrophages infiltrate adipose tissue and secrete a variety of cytokines that cause inflammation, insulin resistance, and predispose to atherosclerotic vascular disease including hypertension, dyslipidemia, type 2 diabetes, and enhanced predisposition to thrombosis. Thus, in obesity it is now possible to evaluate a patient's risk profile for the development of these comorbidities.

There are key hormones produced by adipose tissue, such as leptin, that signal the brain regarding satiety and food intake **(Fig. 2-6)**.

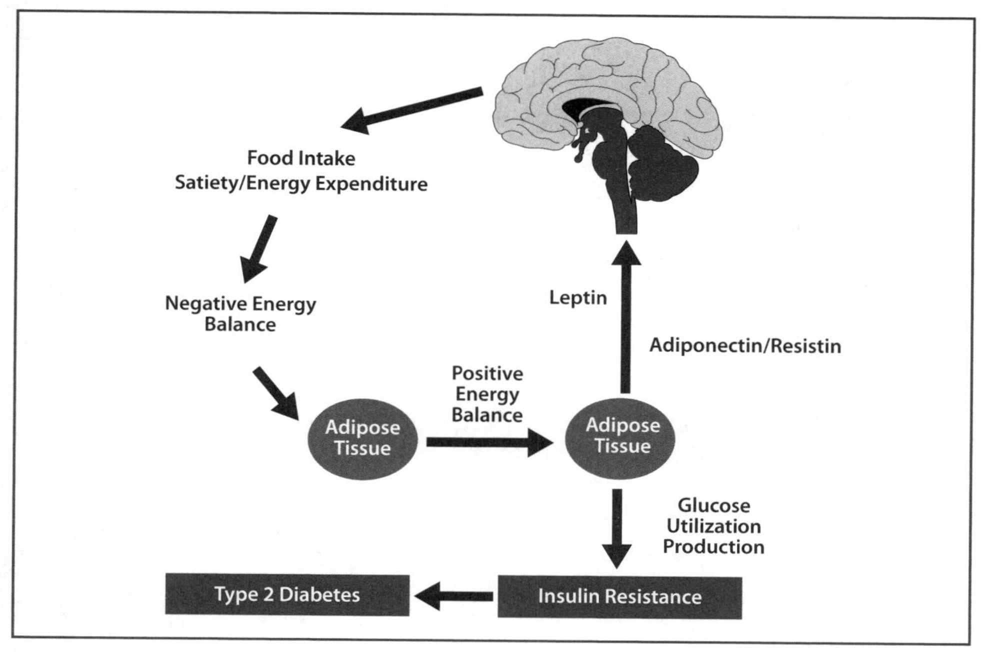

Figure 2-6. Regulation of Food Intake and Energy Balance

Adipose tissue also produces cytokines such as resistin and omentin that increase the resistance to insulin **(Fig. 2-7)**, and the gut produces ghrelin (mostly from the duodenum), which is a satiety signal with receptors in the hypothalamus.

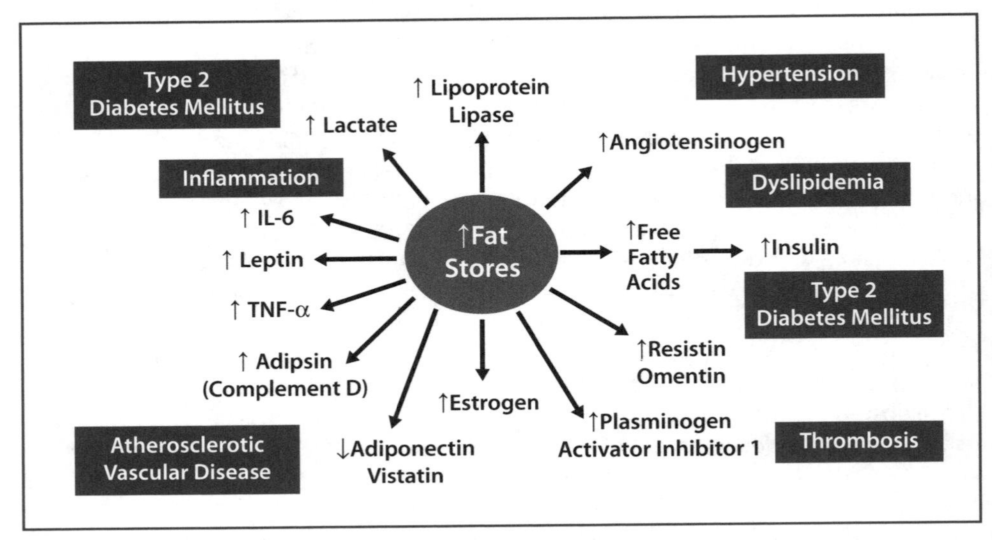

Figure 2-7. Visceral Fat Contributing to the Comorbidities of Obesity

What to Look For

Distinguishing Signs and Symptoms

- BMI >25 (increased risk of morbidity)
- Increased waist circumference (men: >102 cm [>40 in]; women: >88 cm [>36 in])
- Family history of obesity, diabetes, or heart disease
- Evidence of any of the comorbidities listed in Table 2-6
- Risk factor assessment

The Next Step

- Recommend the following measures:
  - Reduced-calorie diet (20% below usual intake)
  - Increased physical activity to improve cardiovascular functions (not likely to reduce weight but has potential to reduce comorbidities)
  - Pharmacological treatments
- Consider bariatric surgery (e.g., gastric bypass in severe obesity [BMI >40])

Table 2-7 provides a diagnostic schema for underlying causes of obesity.

Table 2-7. Diagnostic and Laboratory Evaluation of the Obese Patient Based on Presentation of Symptoms and Risk Factors

For Diagnosis of:	Confirming With:
Alveolar hypoventilation (syndrome, hypersomnolence, possible right-sided heart failure)	• Complete blood count<em>rule out polycythemia • Pulmonary function tests to measure if lung function is reduced • Blood gases<em>measure if CO_2 is elevated • Electrocardiogram<em>rule out right-heart strain
Cushing's syndrome	• 24-Hour urine screen for free cortisol (>150 µg/24 h considered normal) • Overnight DST: 1 mg orally at 11:00 PM. At precisely 8:00 AM the next morning, draw serum cortisol (<5 µg is normal suppression; axis intact). Failure of suppression indicates dysregulation, possibly Cushing's syndrome
Gallstones	• Ultrasonography of gallbladder
Hepatomegaly/nonalcoholic steatohepatitis	• Liver function tests
Hypothyroidism	• Serum TSH (normal <5 µU/mL)
Insulinoma	• Insulin and C-peptide levels will be elevated if insulinoma is present. (Patient should be off insulin and other hyperglycemic drugs for 48 hours prior to test.)
Sleep apnea	• Sleep studies for oxygen desaturation, apneic, and hypopneic events; ear, nose and throat examination for upper airway obstruction
Polycystic ovary syndrome (PCOS; oligomenorrhea, hirsutism, obesity, and enlarged palpable ovaries)	• Increase in LH/FSH ratio, often >2.5. Increased LH stimulates testosterone and androstenedione, converting it to estrone in adipose tissue, leading in turn to increased LH and a continuous cycle.

Modified from Kushner RF, Weinsier RL. Evaluation of the obese patient. Practical considerations. Med Clin North Am. Mar;84(2):387-99, 2000.

ICD-9 CODE: Obesity 278.00

Adrenal 255.8
Due to hyperalimentation 278.00
Endocrine NEC 259.9
Endogenous 259.9
Adiposogential dystrophy 253.8
Glandular NEC 259.9
Hypothyroid 244.9
Morbid 278.01
Of pregnancy 646.1
Severe 278.01
Thyroid 244.9

Reference

1. National Institutes of Health; National Heart, Lung, and Blood Institute in cooperation with the National Institute for Diabetes and Digestive and Kidney Diseases. Clinical guidelines on the identification, evaluation, and treatment of overweight and obesity in adults: the evidence report. NIH pub no. 98-403, 1998. Available at: http://www.nhlbi.nih.gov/guidelines/obesity/ob_gdlns.pdf. Accessed March 1, 2006.

Metabolic Syndrome

The metabolic syndrome is also referred to as dysmetabolic syndrome, syndrome X, insulin resistance syndrome, and multiple metabolic syndrome. It affects 47 million adult Americans, or more than one in five people.

What to Look For

Distinguishing Signs and Symptoms

Obesity, particularly abdominal obesity, is the hallmark of this condition **(Fig. 2-8)**, and is frequently associated with the following conditions:

- Diabetes and hyperglycemia
- Abnormal lipid profile
- Hyperinsulinemia and/or insulin resistance which may promote vascular endothelial dysfunction and hypertension
- Vascular inflammation
- Accelerated cardiovascular disease
- Derangements of adipocyte cytokines

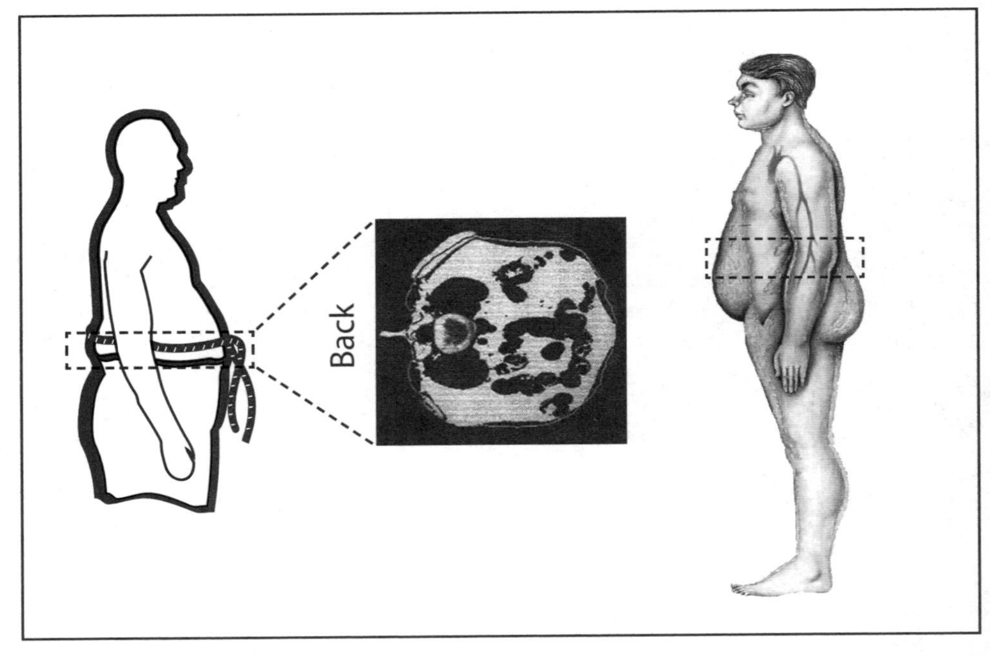

Figure 2-8. Visceral Fat Distribution Seen on Abdominal CT and the Use of a Tape Measure

There are different criteria (Grundy 2004) for the syndrome based on the World Health Organization (WHO), and the National Cholesterol Education recommends the diagnosis be based on the presence of three of the biochemical values noted in **Table 2-8.**

Table 2-8. Diagnostic Criteria for the Dysmetabolic Syndrome: A Comparison of ATPIII and WHO Definitions

Factors for Metabolic Syndrome	ATPIII (3 or More)	Factors for Metabolic Syndrome	WHO (1998) IGT or Insulin Resistance (2 or More)
Abdominal obesity (waist circumference) Men Women	 >102 cm (>40 in) >88 cm (>36 in)	Waist-to-hip ratio Men Women	 >0.8 >0.86 and or BMI > 30 kg/m^2
Triglyceride level	>150 mg/dL		>150 mg/dL
HDL cholesterol level Men Women	<40 mg/dL <50 mg/dL	Men Women	<35 mg/dL <39 mg/dL
Blood pressure	>130/85 mm Hg	Blood Pressure	>160/90 mm Hg or any hypertensive medication
Fasting blood glucose level	>110 mg/dL	Microalbuminuria	>20 µg/min >20 mg/g Cr on at least 2 different occasions

From Brewer HB Jr, Cleeman JI, et al. Definition of metabolic syndrome: report of the National Heart, Lung, and Blood Institute/ American Heart Association conference on scientific issues related to definition. Circulation. Jan 27;109(3):433-8, 2004.

The WHO has a similar definition but requires the sine qua non of an elevated fasting glucose (>110 mg/dL) or a postprandial glucose greater than 200 mg/dL. The American Association of Clinical Endocrinologists proposes a third set of clinical criteria that is a hybrid of the above two but adds age, a family history of vascular disease or diabetes, and inclusion in ethnic groups with a high incidence of diabetes. No defined number of risk factors are specified, rather, identification of the syndrome is left to clinical judgment.

INSULIN RESISTANCE

Insulin resistance cannot simply be defined by the presence of obesity and hyperglycemia, although in practice this is usually the case. Patients with type 1 diabetes or chronic pancreatitis are hyperglycemic but usually do not have insulin resistance, and there are many syndromes associated with extreme insulin resistance that are not associated with obesity. These include inherited lipodystrophies (complete or partial absence of body fat), insulin receptor mutations (leprechaunism), counter-regulatory hormone excess (e.g., glucocorticoids, GH, catecholamines), pregnancy, starvation, kidney failure, and liver failure **(Fig. 2-9)**.

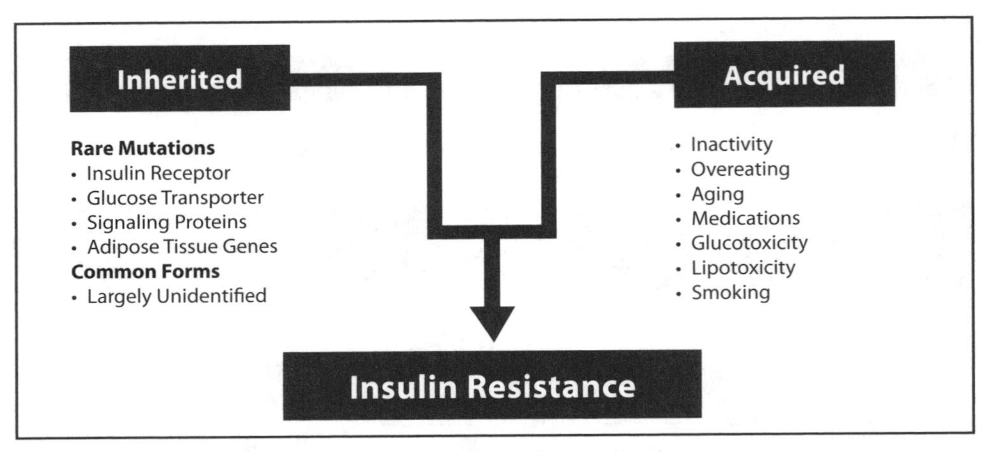

Figure 2-9. Insulin Resistance: Inherited and Acquired Influences

The gold standard for diagnosing insulin resistance is the euglycemic insulin clamp. Insulin-induced glucose uptake is measured while insulin is infused at a constant rate and the blood glucose concentration is kept constant with a variable glucose infusion to avoid the confounding effect of the counter-regulatory hormones glucagons and epinephrine. This procedure allows determination of the rate of maximal glucose uptake under maximal insulin stimulation. Muscle is the organ most responsible for glucose disposal and is believed to be the major tissue responsible for apparent insulin resistance. Because the insulin clamp is a cumbersome and labor-intensive test, it is only used in research settings. The following metabolic markers have been found to correlate with insulin resistance:

- Triglyceride level greater than 150 mg/dL
- Triglyceride/HDL ratio greater than 3
- Fasting serum insulin level greater than 25 μU/mL

Another laboratory test that generally correlates with the insulin clamp technique is the homeostasis model assessment of insulin resistance (HOMA IR). In this test, the product of fasting glucose (in milligrams per deciliter) and fasting insulin (in microunits per milliliter) of <2.77 correlates loosely with insulin insensitivity.

THE NEXT STEP

Initiate lifestyle changes with nutritional therapy, exercise therapy, and appropriate medications to target associate conditions such as dyslipidemia, hyperglycemia, high blood pressure, and cardiovascular disease. Therapy should be tailored to fit individual needs.

ICD-9 CODE: Dysmetabolic Syndrome X 277.7

(See Diabetes Type 2 Screen [Chapter 4] for lipoprotein profile, peptides and cytokines and Oxidative/Nitrosative Stress Profile [Chapter 4] for specific tests and CPT codes)

Reference

1. Grundy SM, Brewer HB Jr, Cleeman JI, et al. Definition of metabolic syndrome: report of the National Heart, Lung, and Blood Institute/American Heart Association conference on scientific issues related to definition. Circulation. Jan 27;109(3):433-8, 2004.

Polycystic Ovary Syndrome

Initially described by Stein and Leventhal (1935) as amenorrhea associated with polycystic ovaries, classic polycystic ovary syndrome (PCOS), which is associated with obesity, acne, and hirsutism in one third of patients, is extremely complex. Two thirds of PCOS patients are not obese, nor are they hirsute. A more functional definition would be chronic, unexplained hyperandrogenism in young women; approximately 95% these patients are diagnosed with PCOS. This definition is more accurate because 50% of patients with PCOS may not have polycystic ovaries or an elevated LH, which were previously part of the diagnostic constellation.

LH excess is postulated to arise from lack of pituitary suppression because of altered sex steroid feedback (increased androgens counteracting the normally suppressive effects of progesterone on LH release). Paradoxically, the more obese the patient, the more likely LH levels will be normal, perhaps related to hyperinsulinism-induced upregulation of ovarian LH receptors.

Infertility and anovulation are not always seen with PCOS, and some patients with obesity and hyperandrogenism are reproductively normal. Patients with PCOS who seek medical attention because of infertility or hirsutism represent only a small proportion of the population with the syndrome.

What to Look For

Distinguishing Signs and Symptoms

- Hirsutism
- Hyperandrogenism
  - Acne
  - Hair loss
- Hyperhidrosis
- Virilization (rare)
- Menstrual irregularity
  - Oligorrhea or amenorrhea
  - Anovulation with infertility
- Obesity
- Insulin resistance
- Acanthosis nigricans (hyperandrogenism, insulin resistance, and acanthosis nigricans [HAIR-AN] syndrome)

Rule out other causes of androgen excess, which may include the following:
- Cushing's syndrome
- Congenital adrenal hyperplasia
- Ovarian and adrenal tumors
- Ovarian hyperthecosis
- Hyperprolactinemia

The Next Step

Hormones and Peptides

- Total and free testosterone
- Sex hormone–binding globulin
- Dehydroepiandrostenedione sulphate
- Prolactin
- TSH
- 17-Alpha-hydroxy progesterone
- Glucose (fasting)
- Insulin
- C-peptide

ICD-9 CODE: PCOS 256.4

ICD-9 CODE: Amenorrhea 626.0
Ovarian dysfunction 256.8
Hyperhormonal 256.8

ICD-9 CODE: Oligomenorrhea 626.1

ICD-9 CODE: Hirsutism 704.1

ICD-9 CODE: Hyperhidrosis 705.21

ICD-9 CODE: Obesity 278.00

ICD-9 CODE: Acanthosis Nigricans 701.2

ICD-9 CODE: Virilization 255.2

(See Polycystic Ovary Syndrome Screen [Chapter 4] for specific tests and CPT codes)

DIABETES MELLITUS

WHAT TO LOOK FOR

Distinguishing Signs and Symptoms

Criteria for the diagnosis of diabetes mellitus are presented in **Table 2-9**.

Table 2-9. Criteria for the Diagnosis of Diabetes Mellitus

1. Symptoms of diabetes plus casual plasma glucose concentration ≥200 mg/dL (11.1 mmol/L). Casual is defined as any time of day without regard to time since last meal. The classic symptoms of diabetes include polyuria, polydipsia, and unexplained weight loss.

OR

2. Fasting plasma glucose ≥126 mg/dL (7.0 mmol/L). Fasting is defined as no caloric intake for at least 8 hours.

OR

3. 2-Hour postload glucose ≥200 mg/dL (11.1 mmol/L) during an oral glucose tolerance test. The test should be performed as described by WHO, using a glucose load containing the equivalent of 75 g anhydrous glucose dissolved in water.

From Genuth S, Alberti KG, Bennett P, et al. Follow-up report on the diagnosis of diabetes mellitus. Diabetes Care. Nov;11:3160-7, 2003.

There are two major forms of diabetes mellitus: type 1 and type 2 **(Table 2-10)**.

Table 2-10. Characteristics of Type 1 and Type 2 Diabetes Mellitus

Characteristic	Type 1	Type 2
Age at diagnosis	<30 years	>30 years
Body weight	Lean	Obese
Family history	Negative	Positive
Insulin level	Absent	Normal/high/low
Ketoacidosis	Prone	Not prone
Hyperosmolar coma	Not prone	Prone
Insulin sensitivity	Sensitive	Resistant
HLA	DR3, DR4	None

Type 1 Diabetes Mellitus

Type 1 diabetes mellitus (previously called juvenile-onset) is characterized by insulin deficiency secondary to the immune destruction of the pancreatic beta cells. The patient cannot survive without exogenous insulin. Other islet cells, including alpha, delta, and PP cells, are normally unaffected. There is a partial genetic link associated with type 1 diabetes, but only about 35% of monozygotic twins share the disorder. Rubella, thyroiditis, and other immunologic disorders tend to coexist with increased incidence of type 1 diabetes. The presence of insulin antibodies and islet cell antibodies are often detected in relatives of patients with type 1 diabetes who subsequently develop the disorder.

Onset can occur soon after birth. However, there is an increase in the onset of type 1 diabetes with the onset of puberty and the development of secondary sexual characteristics. There is a strong association between the histocompatibility (i.e., human leukocyte antigen [HLA]) types and predisposition to and protection from type 1 diabetes **(Fig. 2-10).**

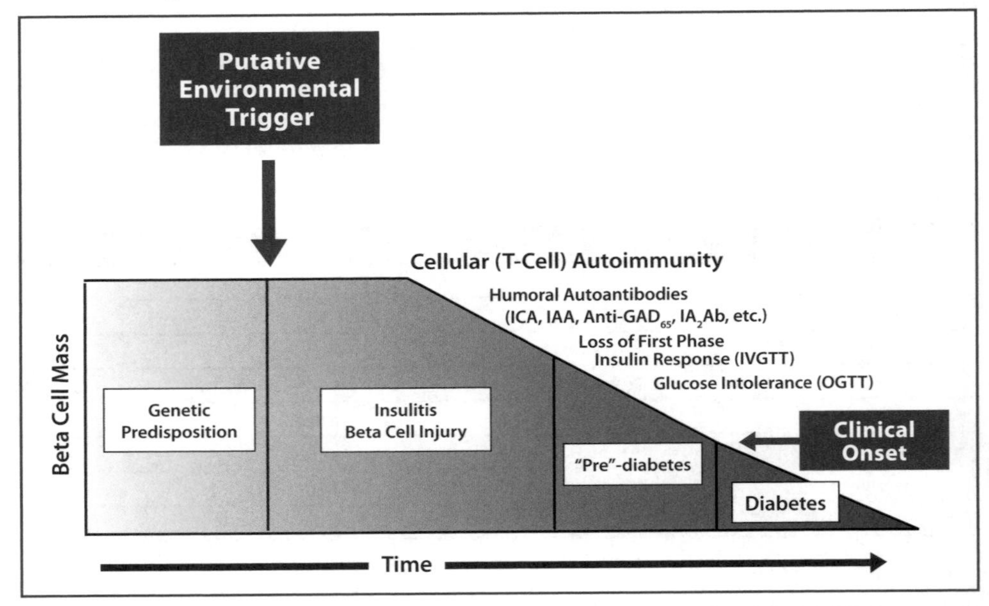

Figure 2-10. The Natural History of Type 1 Diabetes (From Genuth S, Alberti KG, Bennett P, et al. Follow-up report on the diagnosis of diabetes mellitus. *Diabetes Care*. Nov;11:3160-7, 2003.)

- Risk
  - DR3 with DQB1-0201
  - DR4 with DQB1-0302 (2% of the general population and 40% of those with type 1 diabetes have this haplotype)
- Protection
  - DR2 with DQB1-0602

Type 1 diabetes is an autoimmune condition, and a number of molecular antigens have been characterized:

- Insulin autoantibodies (IAA)
- 64-kd Glutamic acid decarboxylase (GAD)
- Milk albumin–related molecule (ICA 69)
- Neuroendocrine tyrosine phosphatase (ICA 512)
- GM2-1 islet ganglioside with terminal sialic acid
- 37- to 40-kd Tryptic fragment of non–GAD 64-kd molecule
- 38-kd T-cell–identified autoantigen

WHAT TO LOOK FOR

Distinguishing Signs and Symptoms

- Polyuria
- Polydypsia
- Ketonuria
- Rapid weight loss

THE NEXT STEP

Hormones and Peptides

Significant hyperglycemia is the primary indicator of type 1 diabetes. It is an autoimmune syndrome superimposed on a genetic susceptibility (HLA DR3 and DR4) and a viral insult resulting in loss of the first phase of insulin secretion in response to intravenous glucose administration culminating in clinical diabetes with greater than 90% destruction of beta cells in the pancreas, loss of insulin secretion, and C-peptide values less than 0.6 ng/mL.

- Measure insulin secretion using the fasting or arginine-stimulated C-peptide level.
- Test for the presence of insulin antibodies that mask insulin production.
- Type for HLA DR3 and DR4 genotype.
- Test for GAD and islet cell, gastric-parietal cell, adrenal, and thyroid antibodies.

Type 1 diabetes is a manageable condition provided detection and treatment are initiated as early as possible. There are many types of insulin delivery systems, including continuous insulin infusion (pumps), daily injections with long- and short-acting insulins mimicking the action of the normal pancreas, as well as inhaled and oral versions of insulin.

ICD-9 CODE: Diabetes Type 1 (Not Stated as Controlled) 250.01

ICD-9 CODE: Diabetes Type 1 (Uncontrolled) 250.03

(See Diabetes Type 1 Screen [Chapter 4] for specific tests and CPT codes)

TYPE 2 DIABETES MELLITUS

Type 2 diabetes is a disorder characterized by diminished liver, muscle, and adipose sensitivity to insulin (insulin resistance) and impaired β-cell function. At the time of diagnosis, most patients with type 2 diabetes present both impaired β-cell function and insulin resistance. It is difficult to determine the primary defect (Burant 2004).

Insulin resistance, which is present, prior to, and early in the development of type 2 diabetes, is frequently found in the relatives of diagnosed type 2 patients, thus providing a means to identify those at risk.

WHAT TO LOOK FOR

Distinguishing Signs and Symptoms

- Polyuria
- Polydipsia
- Fatigue
- Dizziness
- Fasting blood glucose (FBG) greater than 126 mg/dL; 7.0 mmol/L; fasting is defined as no caloric intake for 8 hours)
- Obesity greater than 120% desirable body weight, BMI greater than 27 kg/m^2
- Women with previous gestational diabetes mellitus or history of babies heavier than 9 lbs at birth
- Hypertension or dyslipidemia
- Previously identified impaired glucose tolerance (IGT) or impaired fasting glucose

A complete evaluation should be made to determine the following:

- Type of diabetes
- Presence of underlying diseases requiring further evaluation **(Table 2-11)**
- Presence of complications of diabetes

Table 2-11. Rare Genetic Abnormalities in Diabetes (<0.5% of Type 2 Diabetes Patients)

Condition	Genetic Defect	Frequency
MODY 1	HNF 4a 20q	2%–4% MODY
MODY 2	Glucokinase 7p	11%–63%
MODY 3	HNF1 a Chr 12	21%–73%
MODY 4	Ipf-1/PDX-1	1%–4%
MODY 5	HNF-1b	1%–5%
Maternally-inherited diabetes and deafness	Mitochondrial 3243 tRNA leucine gene	Rare
Mutant insulins	Insulin gene defects	Rare
Defective insulin action	Leprechaunism Rabson-Mendenhall Lipoatrophic diabetes	Rare

THE NEXT STEP

Hormones and Peptides

Hyperinsulinemia is insulin release in response to oral or intravenous glucose.

Who to Test for Asymptomatic Diabetes Mellitus?

- All people over 45 years of age; if negative, repeat tests every 3 years
- Test at younger age if the person has any of the following risk factors:
  - Obesity (body weight >120% or BMI >27 kg/m^2)
  - First-degree relative with type 2 diabetes
  - High-risk population (e.g., African American, American Indians, Hispanic American, Pacific Islander)
  - Hypertension (blood pressure >130/90 mm Hg)
  - HDL <40 mg/dL in males; <50 mg/dL in females
  - Triglycerides >150 mg/dL
  - IGT on a previous test

Figure 2-11 shows the pathogenesis of diabetic macrovascular complications.

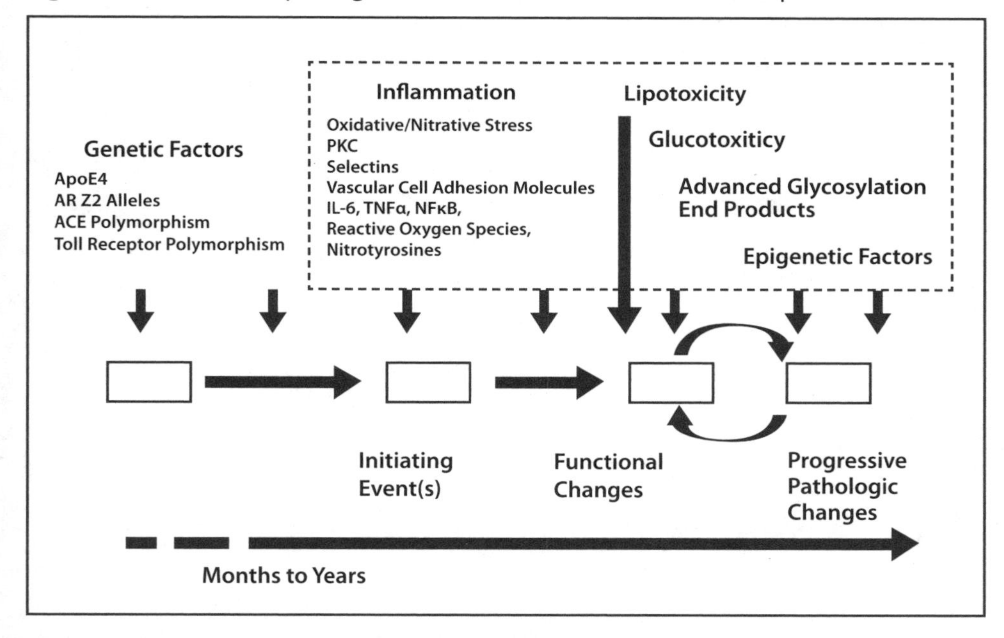

Figure 2-11. Diabetes Disease Initiation/Progression

This schematic suggests the development of microvascular complications early in the course of the disease, well before clinical diabetes is detected. Certain genetic characteristics of polymorphisms (e.g., apolipoprotein E4 (ApoE4), aldose reductase, ACE) may increase an individual's predisposition for development of microvascular complications of diabetes, whereas other genetic factors, such as the toll receptor, are protective and decrease predisposition. The various inflammatory mediators listed under inflammation in Figure 2-11 cause direct cellular injury and initiate the cycle of functional and progressive pathologic changes, which ultimately manifest as microvascular complications. As the disease progresses, lipotoxicity, glucotoxicity, and epigenetic factors further contribute to the functional and pathologic changes. Intervention with insulin or insulin sensitizers, particularly in the early stages of pathogenesis, can counteract inflammatory changes, control glycemia, prevent formation of advanced glycation end products, and ameliorate oxidative stress–induced overactivation of poly adenosine diphosphate ribose polymerase (PARP), with the potential to change the natural history of microvascular complications (Vinik 2004; LeRoith 2004).

ICD-9 CODE: Diabetes Type 2 (Not Stated as Controlled) 250.00

ICD-9 CODE: Diabetes Type 2 (Uncontrolled) 250.02

(See Diabetes Type 2 Screen [Chapter 4] for specific tests and CPT codes)

References

1. Burant CF, ed. ADA Medical Management of Type 2 Diabetes, 5th ed. Alexandria: American Diabetes Association; 2004.
2. Vinik A, Mehrabyan A. Diabetic neuropathies. Med Clin North Am. 88(4):947-99, 2004.
3. LeRoith D, Fonesca V, Vinik A. Metabolic memory in diabetes<em>focus on insulin. Diabetes Metab Res Rev. Mar-Apr;21(2):85-90, 2005.

CELIAC DISEASE

Celiac disease is an autoimmune enteropathy, not an allergy. It is the only autoimmune disease in which the initiating antigen is clearly defined. Celiac disease is also known as celiac sprue, nontropical sprue, and gluten-sensitive enteropathy.

WHAT TO LOOK FOR

Distinguishing Signs and Symptoms

- Symptoms of malabsorption (e.g., weight loss, diarrhea, nutrient deficiencies)
- Occurs mainly in Caucasian children, less often in African-American and Hispanic children
- Osteopenia, bone pain, and pathologic fractures
- Recurrent abdominal pain and/or bloating
- Infertility and/or recurrent miscarriages
- Apthous stomatits
- Diarrhea, weight loss, and failure to thrive
- Fatigue and lassitude
- Depression

Serologic Testing

- Anti–tissue transglutaminase (TTG) immunoglobulin A (IgA) and immunoglobulin G (IgG)
- Antiendomysial IgG and IgA
- Antigliadin IgA and IgG
- Antireticulin antibodies

False-negatives can occur in the following patients:

- Children younger than 2 years of age
- Patients on gluten-free diets for 4 to 6 weeks
- Those with IgA fractions with IgA deficiency (up to 2%–3%)

For a gluten challenge, the patient must ingest three to four slices of wheat bread for 2 to 4 weeks.

False-positives are found in patients with the following conditions:

- Cow's milk protein intolerance
- Parasitic infections (e.g., giardiasis)
- IgA nephropathy
- Crohn's disease
- Eosinophilic gastroenteritis
- Tropical sprue
- Small bowel bacterial overgrowth

Diagnosis of Celiac Disease

- Enzyme found in many tissues; released after injury
- Human-based versus guinea-pig based—Scimedx
- False-positives
- Concurrent autoimmune or inflammatory diseases

- New TTG dot blot test
  - Detects anti-TTG antibodies in serum of 1 drop of whole blood
  - Up to 100% sensitive
  - 96% Specific
  - Takes 30 minutes

Measure the following antibody levels:
- Endomysial (IgA)
- Endomysial titer
- TTG IgG
- TTG IgA

ICD-9 CODE: Celiac Disease 579.0

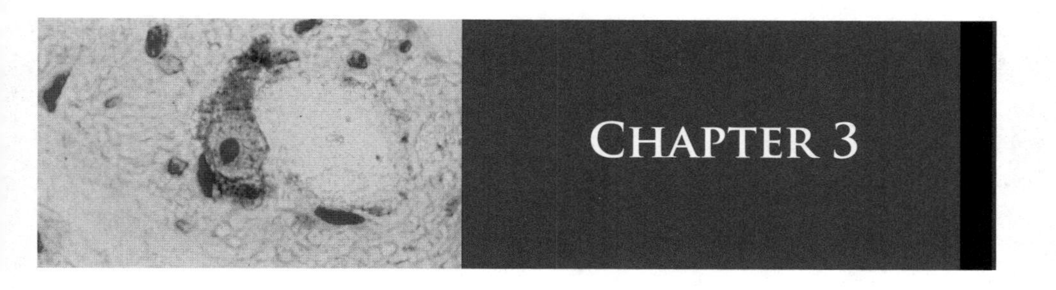

ASSAYS, INCLUDING CPT CODES

INTRODUCTION

PATIENT PREPARATION AND SPECIMEN HANDLING

For **all** tests it is **critical to follow exactly** the specific patient preparation and specimen handling requirements stated for each procedure listed in this catalogue. Factors such as fasting, time of collection, type of specimen, medications used, and method of shipping are vital for obtaining clinically significant information for the appropriate evaluation of a patient. Unless otherwise specified, a morning, fasting specimen is preferred.

Tests that require special preservatives **must** use these special tubes for the collection of specimens to ensure that there is no loss or degradation of the hormone or peptide measured to enable accurate and meaningful determinations of the requested endocrine analytes. Special GI Preservative tubes, TRH preservative tubes and Z-tubes™ are available by request from Inter Science Institute (ISI).

A sample requisition slip is included after the index at the end of this book. Additional requisition slips are available from ISI upon request or directly from the website at interscienceinstitute.com. A requisition slip with the ordering physician's complete address and phone and fax numbers must accompany each specimen. For more information on specific tests or how to obtain appropriate tubes, please call 1-800-255-2873 or email requests to intersci@earthlink.net.

COLLECTION OF SPECIMENS

The majority of hormones are governed by production and clearance rates in blood and urine, which are in dynamic balance in both healthy and disease states. The specific hormone may not be secreted or excreted at a steady rate. Urine tests are requested for various reasons, including eliminating or minimizing the effects of episodic secretion, determining the output of a specific analyte over a full 24-hour period, and obtaining a noninvasive specimen for analysis. The 24-hour urine sampling represents an integrated determination of the individual analytes in question taking into account the production and clearance rates. A random urine specimen is acceptable; however, a 24-hour collection is more readily interpreted within the parameters of the reference range(s).

General Guidelines for Plasma/Serum Specimens

1. Specimens for endocrine procedures preferably should be obtained from patients who have been fasting overnight for 10 to 12 hours.
2. Fasting specimens should be obtained between 6:00 AM and 8:00 AM, unless otherwise stated for a particular procedure.
3. The patient should discontinue medications that may affect hormone levels for at least 48 hours prior to collection under the guidance and consent of their physician (for special instructions see Octreotide [Sandostatin®]).
4. Some tests require the use of the GI preservative collection tube to obtain valid analysis of specimens. Preservative tubes are available from ISI via the internet (intersci@earthlink.net) or via phones: (800) ALL-CURE or (310) 677-3322.
5. Ship specimens frozen via overnight courier service unless otherwise noted under each specific test.

General Guidelines for Collection of a 24-Hour Urine Specimen

1. Begin urine collection after discarding first AM voiding.
2. Collect all other urine voidings during the next 24 hours, including the first AM voiding the next day.
3. Record the 24-hour volume.
4. Mix urine well and remove appropriate aliquot to submit for analysis.
5. Boric acid tablets may be added to urine to reduce bacterial growth.
6. Ensure that urine procedures stating **"Do not acidify urine"** are not collected with hydrochloric or acetic acid.
7. If possible, urine should be refrigerated during collection and shipped frozen to avoid leakage. Provide total volume per 24 hours.
8. Obtain creatinine values for some urine assays (see individual assays listed later in this chapter).

General Guidelines for Collection of a Saliva Specimen

1. Following an overnight fast, saliva should be collected for 5 to 10 minutes.
2. Instruct patient to rinse mouth with water, and wait 10 minutes to begin collecting saliva. Saliva should be allowed to flow freely into container.
3. Instruct the patient to not brush their teeth the morning of collection, because minor abrasions in mouth and/or gingivitis may introduce plasma constituents that affect the level of the hormone being measured.
4. The patient should refrain from intake of food, coffee, and juices for 8 hours prior to collection.
5. The patient should refrain from smoking or chewing gum 8 hours prior to collection.
6. If specimen is collected at home, ensure it is kept refrigerated after collection before transporting to laboratory or physician's office.
7. Record name, date, and beginning time of collection.
8. Have physician's office centrifuge saliva to remove debris before freezing and shipping specimen to ISI.
9. Ship frozen in dry ice.

Fecal Collection

Collect 100 mg (size of dime) of formed stool and store at −20°C. Stool specimens are stable for 7 days when refrigerated. Note on request slip if sample has watery diarrhea consistency, as concentration levels may be decreased due to the dilution factor. See individual tests for additional and specific requirements.

Special Specimens

For tumor/tissue specimens and various fluids (e.g., CSF, peritoneal fluid), see specific test sections or contact ISI for requirements.

Shipping and Instructions

To maintain specimen integrity, ship most specimens frozen in dry ice via an overnight courier such as FedEx® or DHL®. Some specimens are stable at ambient (room) temperature for up to 3 days. See specific tests for stability information and required shipping temperatures.

Contact Information for Inter Science Institute

Phone: (800) 255-2873
Email: intersci@earthlink.net

Some tests listed are in preparation. Contact ISI for availability of tests marked with an asterisk.

ADIPONECTIN*

Reference Range

Reference range is listed on individual patient test reports.

Procedure

Adiponectin is measured by direct radioimmunoassay.

Patient Preparation

The patient should fast for 10 to 12 hours, if possible, prior to collection of specimen. Insulin, medications, or other factors that affect insulin or amylin secretion should be discontinued, if possible, for at least 48 hours prior to collection of specimen.

Specimen Collection

Collect 10 mL of ethylene amine tetraacetic acid (EDTA) plasma in a special tube containing the GI Preservative and separate as soon as possible. Freeze plasma immediately after separation. Special GI Preservative tubes are available from ISI. Minimum specimen size is 1 mL.

Important Precaution

Adiponectin specimens must be collected using the GI Preservative tube. No other methods of collection are acceptable.

Special Specimens

For tumor/tissue and various fluids (e.g., CSF, peritoneal fluid, synovial fluid), contact ISI for requirements and special handling instructions.

Shipping Instructions

Specimens should be shipped frozen in dry ice.

References

1. Fu Y, Luo N, Klein RL, et al. Adiponectin promotes adipocyte differentiation, insulin sensitivity, and lipid accumulation: potential role in autoregulation of adipocyte metabolism and adipose mass. J Lipid Res. July;46(7):1369-79, 2005.
2. Brame LA, Considine RV, Yamauchi M, et al. Insulin and endothelin in the acute regulation of adiponectin in vivo in humans. Obes Res. Mar;13(3):582-8, 2005.
3. Milewicz A, Zatonska K, Demissie M, et al. Serum adiponectin concentration and cardiovascular risk factors in climacteric women. Gynecol Endocrinol. Feb;20(2):68-73, 2005.
4. Ballantyne CM, Nambi V. Markers of inflammation and their clinical significance. Atheroscler Suppl. 2 May;6(2):21-9, 2005.
5. Matsuzawa Y. Adiponectin: identification, physiology and clinical relevance in metabolic and vascular disease. Atheroscler Suppl. May;6(2):7-14, 2005.

*** In preparation**

CPT Code:
Unspecified Quantitative Immunoassay 83519

AMYLIN

Reference Range

Reference range is listed on individual patient test reports.

Procedure

Amylin is measured by direct radioimmunoassay.

Patient Preparation

The patient should fast for 10 to 12 hours, if possible, prior to collection of specimen. Insulin, medications, or other factors that affect insulin or amylin secretion should be discontinued, if possible, for at least 48 hours prior to collection of specimen.

Specimen Collection

Collect 10 mL EDTA plasma in a special tube containing the GI Preservative and separate as soon as possible. Freeze plasma immediately after separation. Special GI Preservative tubes are available from ISI. Minimum specimen size is 1 mL.

Important Precaution

Amylin specimens must be collected using the GI Preservative tube. No other methods of collection are acceptable.

Special Specimens

For tumor/tissue and various fluids (e.g., CSF, peritoneal fluid, synovial fluid), contact ISI for requirements and special handling instructions.

Shipping Instructions

Specimens should be shipped frozen in dry ice.

References

1. Sanke T, Hanabusa T, Nakano Y, et al. Plasma islet amyloid polypeptide (amylin) levels and their responses to oral glucose in type 2 (non-insulin-dependent) diabetic patients. Diabetologia. 34:129-32, 1991.
2. Hartter E, Svoboda T, Lydvik B, et al. Basal and stimulated plasma levels of pancreatic amylin indicate its co-secretion with insulin in humans. Diabetologia. 34:52-4, 1991.
3. Bronsky J, Prusa R. Amylin fasting plasma levels are decreased in patients with osteoporosis. Osteoporos Int. 15(3):243-7, 2004.
4. Samonina GE, Kopylova GN, Lukjanzeva GV, et al. Antiulcer effects of amylin: a review. Pathophysiology. 11(1):1-6, 2004.
5. Ludvik B, Thomaseth K, Nolan JJ, et al. Inverse relation between amylin and glucagon secretion in healthy and diabetic human subjects. Eur J Clin Invest. 33(4):316-22, 2003.

CPT Code:
Unspecified Quantitative Immunoassay 83519

BOMBESIN/GASTRIN-RELEASING PEPTIDE (GRP)

Reference Range

50–250 pg/mL

Procedure

Bombesin is measured by direct radioimmunoassay.

Patient Preparation

The patient should fast for 10 to 12 hours prior to collection of specimen. Antacid medications and medications that affect intestinal motility should be discontinued, if possible, for at least 48 hours prior to collection of specimen.

Specimen Requirements

Collect 10 mL EDTA plasma in a special tube containing the GI Preservative and separate as soon as possible. Freeze plasma immediately after separation. Special GI Preservative tubes are available from ISI. Minimum specimen size is 1 mL.

Important Precaution

Bombesin specimens must be collected using the GI Preservative tube. No other specimens are acceptable.

Special Specimens

For tumor/tissue and various fluids (e.g., CSF, peritoneal fluid, synovial fluid), contact ISI for requirements and special handling instructions.

Shipping Instructions

Specimens should be shipped frozen in dry ice.

References

1. Mahmoud S, Palaszynski E, Fiskum G, et al. Small cell lung cancer bombesin receptors are antagonized by reduced peptide analogues. Life Sci. 44(5):367-73, 1989.
2. Tache Y, Gunion M. Central nervous system action of bombesin to inhibit gastrin acid secretion. Life Sci. 15 Jul;37(2):115-23, 1985.
3. Yegen BC. Bombesin-like peptides: candidates as diagnostic and therapeutic tools. Curr Pharm. Dec;9(12):1013-22, 2003.
4. Zhou J, Chen J, Mokotoff M, et al. Bombesin/gastrin-releasing peptide receptor: a potential target for antibody-mediated therapy of small cell lung cancer. Clin Cancer Res. 9(13):4953-60, 2003.
5. Mandragos C, Moukas M, Amygdalou A, et al. Gastrointestinal hormones and short-term nutritional schedules in critically ill patients. Hepatogastroenterology. 50(53):1442-5, 2003.
6. Scott N, Millward E, Cartwright EJ, et al. Gastrin releasing peptide and gastrin releasing peptide receptor expression in gastrointestinal carcinoid tumours. J Clin Pathol. 57(2):189-92, 2004.

CPT Code:
Unspecified Quantitative Immunoassay 83519

BRAIN NATRIURETIC PEPTIDE (BNP)*

Reference Range

Reference range is listed on individual patient test reports.

Procedure

BNP is measured by direct radioimmunoassay.

Patient Preparation

The patient should fast for 10 to 12 hours, if possible, prior to collection of specimen. Insulin, medications, or other factors that affect insulin or BNP secretion should be discontinued, if possible, for at least 48 hours prior to collection of specimen.

Specimen Collection

Collect 10 mL EDTA plasma in a special tube containing the GI Preservative and separate as soon as possible. Freeze plasma immediately after separation. Special GI Preservative tubes are available from ISI. Minimum specimen size is 1 mL.

Important Precaution

BNP specimens must be collected using the GI Preservative tube. No other methods of collection are acceptable.

Special Specimens

For tumor/tissue and various fluids (e.g., CSF, peritoneal fluid, synovial fluid), contact ISI for requirements and special handling instructions.

Shipping Instructions

Specimens should be shipped frozen in dry ice.

References

1. Fang ZY, Schull-Meade R, Leano R, et al. Screening for heart disease in diabetic subjects. Am Heart J. Feb;149(2):349-54, 2005.
2. Dokainish H, Zoghbi WA, Lakkis NM, et al. Incremental predictive power of B-type natriuretic peptide and tissue Doppler echocardiography in the prognosis of patients with congestive heart failure. J Am Coll Cardiol. 19 Apr;45(8):1223-6, 2005.
3. Mueller T, Gegenhuber A, Poelz W, et al. Diagnostic accuracy of B type natriuretic peptide and amino terminal proBNP in the emergency diagnosis of heart failure. Heart. May;91(5):606-12, 2005.
4. Mazzone M, Forte P, Portale G, et al. Brain natriuretic peptide and acute coronary syndrome. Minerva Med. Feb;96(1):11-8, 2005.

*** In preparation**

CPT Code:
Brain Natriuretic Peptide (BNP) 83880

C-Peptide

Reference Range

0.9–4.2 ng/mL
Reference range is listed on individual patient test reports.

Procedure

C-peptide is measured by direct radioimmunoassay.

Patient Preparation

The patient should not be on any insulin therapy nor take medications that influence insulin levels, if possible, for at least 48 hours prior to collection of specimen.

Specimen Collection

Collect 3 mL of serum or EDTA plasma and separate as soon as possible. Freeze serum or plasma immediately after separation. Minimum specimen size is 1 mL.

Special Specimens

For tumor/tissue and various fluids (e.g., CSF, peritoneal fluid, synovial fluid), contact ISI for requirements and special handling instructions.

Shipping Instructions

Specimens should be shipped frozen in dry ice.

References

1. Myrick JE, Gunter EW, Maggio VL, et al. An improved radioimmunoassay of C-peptide and its application in a multiyear study. Clin Chem. 35:7-42, 1989.
2. Ludvigsson J. Methodological aspects of C-peptide measurements. Acta Med Scand (Suppl). 671:53-9, 1983.
3. Bell DS, Ovalle F. The role of C-peptide levels in screening for latent autoimmune diabetes in adults. Am J Ther. 11(4):308-11, 2004.
4. Jazet IM, Pijl H, Frolich M, et al. Factors predicting the blood glucose lowering effect of a 30-day very low calorie diet in obese type 2 diabetic patients. Diabet Med. 22(1):52-5, 2005.
5. Ovalle F, Bell DS. Effect of rosiglitazone versus insulin on the pancreatic beta-cell function of subjects with type 2 diabetes. Diabetes Care. 27(11):2585-9, 2005.
6. Landin-Olsson M. Latent autoimmune diabetes in adults. Ann NY Acad Sci. Apr;958:112-6, 2002.
7. Torn C. C-peptide and autoimmune markers in diabetes. Clin Lab. 49(1-2):1-10, 2003.

CPT Codes:
C-Peptide 80432, 84681

C-REACTIVE PROTEIN (CRP; HIGHLY SENSITIVE FOR METABOLIC SYNDROME)*

Reference Range

Reference range is listed on individual patient test reports.

Procedure

CRP is measured by direct radioimmunoassay.

Patient Preparation

The patient should fast for 10 to 12 hours prior to collection of specimen. Antacid medications and medications that affect intestinal motility should be discontinued, if possible, for at least 48 hours prior to collection of specimen.

Specimen Collection

Collect 10 mL EDTA plasma in a special tube containing the GI Preservative and separate as soon as possible. Freeze plasma immediately after separation. Special GI Preservative tubes are available from ISI. Minimum specimen size is 1 mL.

Important Precaution

CRP specimens must be collected using the GI Preservative tube. No other specimens are acceptable.

Special Specimens

For tumor/tissue and various fluids (e.g., CSF, peritoneal fluid, synovial fluid), contact ISI for requirements and special handling instructions.

Shipping Instructions

Specimens should be shipped frozen in dry ice.

Reference

1. Valle M, Martos R, Gascon F, et al. Low-grade systemic inflammation, hypoadiponectinemia and a high concentration of leptin are present in very young obese children, and correlate with metabolic syndrome. Diabetes Metab. Feb;31(1):55-62, 2005.

*** In preparation**

CPT Codes:
C-Reactive Protein (Inflammation and CSF) 86140
C-Reactive Protein (Cardiac Risk) 86141

C-REACTIVE PROTEIN (CRP; REGULAR FOR INFLAMMATION)*

Reference Range

Reference range is listed on individual patient test reports.

Procedure

CRP is measured by direct radioimmunoassay.

Patient Preparation

The patient should fast for 10 to 12 hours prior to collection of specimen. Antacid medications and medications that affect intestinal motility should be discontinued, if possible, for at least 48 hours prior to collection of specimen.

Specimen Collection

Collect 10 mL EDTA plasma in a special tube containing the GI Preservative and separate as soon as possible. Freeze plasma immediately after separation. Special GI Preservative tubes are available from ISI. Minimum specimen size is 1 mL.

Important Precaution

CRP specimens must be collected using the GI Preservative tube. No other specimens are acceptable.

Special Specimens

For tumor/tissue and various fluids (e.g., CSF, peritoneal fluid, synovial fluid), contact ISI for requirements and special handling instructions.

Shipping Instructions

Specimens should be shipped frozen in dry ice.

Reference

1. Valle M, Martos R, Gascon F, et al. Low-grade systemic inflammation, hypoadiponectinemia and a high concentration of leptin are present in very young obese children, and correlate with metabolic syndrome. Diabetes Metab. Feb;31(1):55-62, 2005.

*** In preparation**

CPT Codes:
C-Reactive Protein (Inflammation and CSF) 86140
C-Reactive Protein (Cardiac Risk) 86141

CALCITONIN (THYROCALCITONIN)

Reference Range

Up to 300 pg/mL
Reference range is listed on individual patient test reports.

Procedure

Calcitonin is measured by direct radioimmunoassay.

Patient Preparation

The patient should fast for 10 to 12 hours prior to collection of specimen. Thyroid medications and medications that affect intestinal motility should be discontinued, if possible, for at least 48 hours prior to collection of specimen.

Specimen Collection

Collect 3 mL serum or EDTA plasma and separate as soon as possible. Freeze serum or plasma immediately after separation. Minimum specimen size is 1 mL.

Special Specimens

For tumor/tissue and various fluids (e.g., CSF, peritoneal fluid, synovial fluid), contact ISI for requirements and special handling instructions.

Shipping Instructions

Specimens should be shipped frozen in dry ice.

References

1. Kempter B, Ritter MM. Unexpected high calcitonin concentrations after pentagastrin stimulation. Clin Chem. Mar;37(3):473-4, 1991.
2. Hurley DL, Tiegs RD, Wahner H, et al. Axial and appendicular bone mineral density in patients with long-term deficiency or excess of calcitonin. N Engl J Med. 27 Aug;317(9):537-41, 1987.

CPT Code:
Calcitonin 82308

CARBOXY METHYL LYSINE (CML)*

Reference Range

Up to 80 pg/mL
Reference range is listed on individual patient test reports.

Procedure

CML is measured by direct radioimmunoassay.

Patient Preparation

The patient should fast for 10 to 12 hours prior to collection of specimen. Antacid medications and medications that affect intestinal motility should be discontinued, if possible, for at least 48 hours prior to collection of specimen.

Specimen Collection

Collect 10 mL EDTA plasma in a special tube containing the GI Preservative and separate as soon as possible. Freeze plasma immediately after separation. Special GI Preservative tubes are available from ISI. Minimum specimen size is 1 mL.

Important Precaution

CML specimens must be collected using the GI Preservative tube. No other specimens are acceptable.

Special Specimens

For tumor/tissue and various fluids (e.g., CSF, peritoneal fluid, synovial fluid), contact ISI for requirements and special handling instructions.

Shipping Instructions

Specimens should be shipped frozen in dry ice.

References

1. Hirata K, Kubo K. Relationship between blood levels of N-carboxymethyl-lysine and pentosidine and the severity of microangiopathy in type 2 diabetes. Endocr J. Dec;51(6):537-44, 2004.
2. Petrovic R, Futas J, Chandoga J, et al. Rapid and simple method for determination of N(epsilon)-(carboxymethyl)lysine and N(epsilon)-(carboxyethyl)lysine in urine using gas chromatography/mass spectrometry. Biomed Chromatogr. Nov;19(9):649-54, 2005.

*** In preparation**

CPT Code:
Unspecified Quantitative Immunoassay 83519

CHOLECYSTOKININ (CCK)

Reference Range

Up to 80 pg/mL

Procedure

CCK is measured by direct radioimmunoassay.

Patient Preparation

The patient should fast for 10 to 12 hours prior to collection of specimen. Antacid medications and medications that affect intestinal motility should be discontinued, if possible, for at least 48 hours prior to collection of specimen.

Specimen Collection

Collect 10 mL EDTA plasma in a special tube containing the GI Preservative and separate as soon as possible. Freeze plasma immediately after separation. Special GI Preservative tubes are available from ISI. Minimum specimen size is 1 mL.

Important Precaution

CCK specimens must be collected using the GI Preservative tube. No other specimens are acceptable.

Special Specimens

For tumor/tissue and various fluids (e.g., CSF, peritoneal fluid, synovial fluid), contact ISI for requirements and special handling instructions.

Shipping Instructions

Specimens should be shipped frozen in dry ice.

References

1. Nakano I, Funakoshi A, Shinozaki H, et al. Plasma cholecystokinin and pancreatic polypeptide responses after ingestion of a liquid test meal rich in medium-chain fatty acids in patients with chronic pancreatitis. Am J Clin Nutr. Feb;49(2):247-51, 1989.
2. Chang T, Chey WY. Radioimmunoassay of cholecystokinin. Dig Dis Sci. May;28(5):456-68, 1983.
3. Rehfeld JF. Clinical endocrinology and metabolism. Cholecystokinin. Best Pract Res Clin Endocrinol Metab. 18(4):569-86, 2004.

CPT Code:
Unspecified Quantitative Immunoassay 83519

CHROMOGRANIN A (CgA)

Reference Range

6.0–40.0 ng/mL

Procedure

CgA is measured by direct radioimmunoassay/enzyme immunoassay (EIA)/ELISA.

Patient Preparation

The patient should fast for 10 to 12 hours prior to collection of specimen. Antacid medications and medications that affect intestinal motility should be discontinued, if possible, for at least 48 hours prior to collection of specimen.

Specimen Collection

Collect 10 mL whole blood in an EDTA or red-topped tube. Plasma or serum should be separated as soon as possible. CgA is stable at room temperature for 3 days. Specimen can be stored at ambient temperature, refrigerated, or frozen in dry ice.

Important Precaution

Draw sample first thing in the morning because of the diurnal variation. When serial measurements are made, draw samples at the same time each day.

Shipping Instructions

Specimens can be shipped at ambient temperature, refrigerated, or frozen in dry ice.

References

1. Öberg K, Kvols L, Caplin M, et al. Consensus report on the use of somatostatin analogs for the management of neuroendocrine tumors of the gastroenteropancreatic system. Ann Oncol. 15:966-73, 2004.
2. Nehar D, Olivieri S, Claustrat B, et al. Interest of Chromogranin A for diagnosis and follow-up of endocrine tumours. Clin Endocrinol (Oxf). 60(5):644-52, 2004.
3. Viola KV, Sosa JA. Current advances in the diagnosis and treatment of pancreatic endocrine tumors. Curr Opin Oncol. 17(1):24-7, 2005.
4. d'Herbomez M, Gouze V, Huglo D, et al. Chromogranin A assay and 131I-MIBG scintigraphy for diagnosis and follow-up of pheochromocytoma. J Nucl Med. Jul;42(7):993-7, 2001.
5. Giusti M, Sidoti M, Augeri C, et al. Effect of short-term treatment with low dosages of the proton-pump inhibitor omeprazole on serum chromogranin A levels in man. Eur J Endocrinol. Mar;150(3):299-303, 2004.
6. Biausque F, Jaboureck O, Devos P, et al. Clinical significant of serum chromogranin A levels for diagnosing pheochromocytoma in hypertensive patients. Arch Mal Coeur Vaiss. Jul-Aug;96(7-8):780-3, 2003.
7. Giampaolo B, Angelica M, Antonio S. Chromogranin 'A' in normal subjects, essential hypertensives and adrenalectomized patients. Clin Endocrinol. Jul;57(1):41-50, 2002.

CPT Code:
Unspecified Quantitative Immunoassay 86316

Elastase, Pancreatic, Serum

Reference Range

30–125 ng/mL
Reference range is listed on individual patient test reports.

Procedure

Elastase is measured by direct radioimmunoassay.

Patient Preparation

The patient should fast for 10 to 12 hours prior to collection of specimen. Medications that affect pancreatic activity should be discontinued, if possible, for at least 48 hours prior to collection of specimen.

Specimen Collection

Collect 3 mL serum and separate as soon as possible. Freeze serum immediately after separation. Minimum specimen size is 1 mL.

Special Specimens

For tumor/tissue and various fluids (e.g., CSF, peritoneal fluid, synovial fluid), contact ISI for requirements and special handling instructions.

Shipping Instructions

Specimens should be shipped frozen in dry ice.

References

1. Wortsman J, Matsuoka LY, Kueppers F. Elastase inhibitory activity in serum of patients with thyroid dysfunction. Clin Chem. 37:108-10, 1991.
2. Geokas MC, Brodrick JW, Johnson JH, et al. Pancreatic elastase in human serum. Determination by radioimmunoassay. J Biol Chem. 10 Jan; 252(1):61-7, 1977.

CPT Code:
Pancreatic Elastase I 82656

ELASTASE-1 (EL1), FECAL

Reference Ranges

Normal: 200 to >500 μg/g stool
Moderate to mild pancreatic insufficiency: 100–200 μg/g stool
Severe exocrine pancreatic insufficiency: <100 μg/g stool

Procedure

EL1 is measured by a monoclonal antibody specific only to human pancreatic EL1 employing ELISA.

Patient Preparation

No special patient preparation is required, because substitution therapy has no influence on the specific fecal EL1 levels.

Specimen Collection

Collect 100 mg formed stool and store at −20°C. Stool specimens are stable for 7 days when refrigerated. Minimum specimen size is 20 mg of formed stool. Note if sample has watery diarrhea consistency, as the concentration of EL1 may be decreased due to the dilution factor.

Special Specimens

Stool is the only appropriate specimen for this test (see Elastase, Pancreatic, Serum).

Shipping Instructions

Specimens should be shipped frozen in dry ice.

References

1. Hahn JU, Bochnig S, Kerner W, et al. A new fecal elastase 1 test using polyclonal antibodies for the detection of exocrine pancreatic insufficiency. Pancreas. Mar;30(2):189-91, 2005.
2. Luth S, Teyssen S, Forssmann K, et al. Fecal elastase-1 determination: 'gold standard' of indirect pancreatic function tests? Scand J Gastroenterol. Oct;36(10):1092-9, 2001.
3. Gullo L, Ventrucci M, Tomassetti P, et al. Fecal elastase 1 determination in chronic pancreatitis. Dig Dis Sci. Jan;44(1):210-3, 1999.

CPT Code:
Fecal Elastase 82656

Exendin*

Reference Range

Reference range is listed on individual patient test reports.

Procedure

Exendin is measured by direct radioimmunoassay.

Patient Preparation

The patient should fast for 10 to 12 hours prior to collection of specimen. Medications that affect pancreatic activity should be discontinued, if possible, for at least 48 hours prior to collection of specimen.

Specimen Collection

Collect 3 mL serum or EDTA plasma and separate as soon as possible. Freeze serum or plasma immediately after separation. Minimum specimen size is 1 mL.

Special Specimens

For tumor/tissue and various fluids (e.g., CSF, peritoneal fluid, synovial fluid), contact ISI for requirements and special handling instructions.

Shipping Instructions

Specimens should be shipped frozen in dry ice.

References

1. Hansen PA, Corbett JA. Incretin hormones and insulin sensitivity. Trends Endocrinol Metab. May-Jun;16(4):135-6, 2005.
2. Calara F, Taylor K, Han J, et al. A randomized, open-label, crossover study examining the effect of injection site on bioavailability of exenatide (synthetic exendin-4). Clin Ther. Feb;27(2):210-5, 2005.
3. Dupre J. Glycaemic effects of incretins in type 1 diabetes mellitus: a concise review, with emphasis on studies in humans. Regul Pept. 15 Jun;128(2):149-57, 2005.

*** In preparation**

CPT Code:
Unspecified Quantitative Immunoassay 83519

FIBRINOGEN*

Reference Range

Reference range is listed on individual patient test reports.

Procedure

Fibrinogen is measured by direct radioimmunoassay.

Patient Preparation

The patient should fast for 10 to 12 hours prior to collection of specimen. Medications that affect pancreatic activity should be discontinued, if possible, for at least 48 hours prior to collection of specimen.

Specimen Collection

Collect 3 mL serum or EDTA plasma and separate as soon as possible. Freeze serum or plasma immediately after separation. Minimum specimen size is 1 mL.

Special Specimens

For tumor/tissue and various fluids (e.g., CSF, peritoneal fluid, synovial fluid), contact ISI for requirements and special handling instructions.

Shipping Instructions

Specimens should be shipped frozen in dry ice.

Reference

1. Please refer to www.endotext.org.

*** In preparation**

CPT Codes:
Fibrinogen 85384–85385

Galanin

Reference Range

25–80 pg/mL
Reference range is listed on individual patient test reports.

Procedure

Galanin is measured by direct radioimmunoassay.

Patient Preparation

The patient should fast for 10 to 12 hours prior to collection of specimen. Medications that affect intestinal motility or insulin levels should be discontinued, if possible, for at least 48 hours prior to collection of specimen.

Specimen Collection

Collect 10 mL EDTA plasma in a special tube containing the GI Preservative and separate as soon as possible. Freeze plasma immediately after separation. Special GI Preservative tubes are available from ISI. Minimum specimen size is 1 mL.

Important Precaution

Galanin specimens must be collected using the GI Preservative tube. No other specimens are acceptable.

Special Specimens

For tumor/tissue and various fluids (e.g., CSF, peritoneal fluid, synovial fluid) contact ISI for requirements and special handling instructions.

Shipping Instructions

Specimens should be shipped frozen in dry ice.

References

1. Nilsson T, Arkhammar P, Rorsman P, et al. Suppression of insulin release by galanin and somatostatin is mediated by a G-Protein. J Biol Chem. 264:973-80, 1989.
2. Tatemoto K, Rokaeus A, Jornvall H, et al. Galanin—a novel biologically active peptide from porcine intestine. FEBS Lett. 28 Nov;164(1):124-8, 1983.
3. Basuyau JP, Mallet E, Leroy M, et al. Reference intervals for serum calcitonin in men, women, and children. Clin Chem. 50(10):1828-30, 2004.
4. Gimm O, Ukkat J, Niederle BE, et al. Timing and extent of surgery in patients with familial medullary thyroid carcinoma/multiple endocrine neoplasia 2A-related RET mutations not affecting codon 634. World J Surg. 28(12):1312-6, 2004.
5. Harmar AJ. Clinical endocrinology and metabolism. Receptors for gut peptides. Best Pract Res Clin Endocrinol Metab. 18(4):463-75, 2004.

CPT Code:
Unspecified Quantitative Immunoassay 83519

GASTRIC INHIBITORY POLYPEPTIDE (GIP; GLUCOSE-DEPENDENT INSULINOTROPIC PEPTIDE)

Reference Range

75–325 pg/mL
Reference range is listed on individual patient test reports.

Procedure

GIP is measured by direct radioimmunoassay.

Patient Preparation

The patient should fast for 10 to 12 hours prior to collection of specimen. Antacid medications and medications that affect intestinal motility or insulin secretion should be discontinued, if possible, for at least 48 hours prior to collection of specimen.

Specimen Collection

Collect 10 mL EDTA plasma in a special tube containing the GI Preservative and separate as soon as possible. Freeze plasma immediately after separation. Special GI Preservative tubes are available from ISI. Minimum specimen size is 1 mL.

Important Precaution

GIP specimens must be collected using the GI Preservative tube. No other specimens are acceptable.

Special Specimens

For tumor/tissue and various fluids (e.g., CSF, peritoneal fluid, synovial fluid) contact ISI for requirements and special handling instructions.

Shipping Instructions

Specimens should be shipped frozen in dry ice.

References

1. Krarup T. Immunoreactive gastric inhibitory polypeptide. Endocr Rev. Feb;9(1):122-34, 1988.
2. Sarson DL, Bryant MG, Bloom SR. A radioimmunoassay of gastric inhibitory polypeptide in human plasma. J Endocrinol. Jun;85(3):487-96, 1980.
3. Thomas RP, Hellmich MR, Townsend CM Jr, et al. Role of gastrointestinal hormones in the proliferation of normal and neoplastic tissues. Endocr Rev. 24(5):571-99, 2003.
4. Calhoun K, Toth-Fejel S, Cheek J, et al. Serum peptide profiles in patients with carcinoid tumors. Am J Surg. 186(1): 28-3, 2003.
5. Meier JJ, Nauck, MA. Clinical endocrinology and metabolism. Glucose-dependent insulinotropic polypeptide/gastric inhibitory polypeptide. Best Pract Res Clin Endocrinol Metab. 18(4):587-606, 2004.
6. Nauck MA, Baller B, Meier JJ. Gastric inhibitory polypeptide and glucagon-like peptide-1 in the pathogenesis of type 2 diabetes. Diabetes. 53(Suppl 3):S190-6, 2004.

CPT Code:
Unspecified Quantitative Immunoassay 83519

Gastrin

Reference Range

0–100 pg/mL
Reference range is listed on individual patient test reports.

Procedure

Gastrin is measured by direct radioimmunoassay.

Patient Preparation

The patient should fast for 10 to 12 hours prior to collection of specimen. Antacid medications should be discontinued, if possible, for at least 48 hours prior to collection of specimen.

Specimen Collection

Collect 3 mL serum or EDTA plasma and separate as soon as possible. Freeze serum or plasma immediately after separation. Minimum specimen size is 1 mL.

Special Specimens

For tumor/tissue and various fluids (e.g., CSF, peritoneal fluid, synovial fluid) contact ISI for requirements and special handling instructions.

Shipping Instructions

Specimens should be shipped frozen in dry ice.

References

1. Bostwick DG, Bensch KG. Gastrin releasing peptide in human neuroendocrine tumors. J Pathol. Dec;147(4):237-44, 1985.
2. Walsh JH, Isenberg JI, Ansfield J, et al. Clearance and acid-stimulating action of human big and little gastrins in duodenal ulcer subjects. J Clin Invest. May;57(5):1125-31, 1976.
3. Dockray G, Dimaline R, Varro A. Gastrin: old hormone, new functions. Pflugers Arch. 449(4): 344-55, 2005.
4. Mignon, M. Diagnostic and therapeutic strategies in Zollinger-Ellison syndrome associated with multiple endocrine neoplasia type I (MEN-I): experience of the Zollinger-Ellison Syndrome Research Group: Bichat 1958-1999. Bull Acad Nat Med. 187(7):1249-58, 2003.

CPT Codes:
Gastrin 82938–82941

GASTRIN-RELEASING PEPTIDE (GRP; BOMBESIN)

Reference Range

10–80 pg/mL
Reference range is listed on individual patient test reports.

Procedure

GRP is measured by direct radioimmunoassay.

Patient Preparation

The patient should fast for 10 to 12 hours prior to collection of specimen. Antacid medications and medications that affect intestinal motility should be discontinued, if possible, for at least 48 hours prior to collection of specimen.

Specimen Collection

Collect 10 mL EDTA plasma in a special tube containing the GI Preservative and separate as soon as possible. Freeze plasma immediately after separation. Special GI Preservative tubes are available from ISI. Minimum specimen size is 1 mL.

Important Precaution

GRP specimens must be collected using the GI Preservative tube. No other specimens are acceptable.

Special Specimens

For tumor/tissue and various fluids (e.g., CSF, peritoneal fluid, synovial fluid) contact ISI for requirements and special handling instructions.

Shipping Instructions

Specimens should be shipped frozen in dry ice.

References

1. Bostwick DG, Bensch KG. Gastrin releasing peptide in human neuroendocrine tumors. J Pathol. Dec;147(4):237-44, 1985.
2. Carney DN, Cuttitta F, Moody TW, et al. Selective stimulation of small cell lung cancer clonal growth by bombesin and gastrin releasing peptide. Cancer Res. 1 Feb;47(3):821-5, 1987.
3. Thomas RP, Hellmich MR, Townsend CM Jr, et al. Role of gastrointestinal hormones in the proliferation of normal and neoplastic tissues. Endocr Rev. 24(5):571-99, 2003.
4. Calhoun K, Toth-Fejel S, Cheek J, et al. Serum peptide profiles in patients with carcinoid tumors. Am J Surg. 186(1): 28-31, 2003.
5. Sunday ME. Pulmonary neuroendocrine cells and lung development. Endocr Pathol. 7(3):173-201, 1996.

CPT Code:
Unspecified Quantitative Immunoassay 83519

GLUCAGON

Reference Ranges

Age (y)	Range (pg/mL)
20–29	20–180
30–39	10–250
40–49	40–215
50–59	75–170
60–69	50–270

Reference range is listed on individual patient test reports.

Procedure

Glucagon is measured by direct radioimmunoassay.

Patient Preparation

The patient should fast for 10 to 12 hours prior to collection of specimen. The patient should not take any medications that influence insulin secretion or intestinal motility, if possible, for at least 48 hours prior to collection of specimen.

Specimen Collection

Collect 10 mL EDTA plasma and separate immediately. Freeze plasma immediately after separation. Minimum specimen size is 1 mL.

Special Specimens

For tumor/tissue and various fluids (e.g., CSF, peritoneal fluid, synovial fluid) contact ISI for requirements and special handling instructions.

Shipping Instructions

Specimens should be shipped frozen in dry ice.

References

1. Philippe J, Mojsov S, Drucker DJ, et al. Proglucagon processing in a rat islet cell line resembles phenotype of intestine rather than pancreas. Endocrinology. Dec;119(6):2833-9, 1986.
2. Weir GC, Mojsov S, Hendrick GK, et al. Glucagonlike peptide I (7-37) actions on endocrine pancreas. Diabetes. Mar;38(3):338-42, 1989.
3. van Beek AP, de Haas ER, van Vloten WA, et al. The glucagonoma syndrome and necrolytic migratory erythema: a clinical review. Eur J Endocrinol. 151(5):531-7, 2004.

CPT Codes:

Glucagon 82943
- Tolerance Panel 80422–80424
- Tolerance Test 82946

GLUCAGON-LIKE PEPTIDE 1 (GLP-1)

Reference Range

Reference range is listed on individual patient test reports.

Procedure

GLP-1 is measured by direct radioimmunoassay.

Patient Preparation

The patient should fast for 10 to 12 hours prior to collection of specimen. Antacid medications and medications that affect intestinal motility or insulin secretion should be discontinued, if possible, for at least 48 hours prior to collection of specimen.

Specimen Collection

Collect 10 mL EDTA plasma in a special tube containing the GI Preservative and separate as soon as possible. Freeze plasma immediately after separation. Special GI Preservative tubes are available from ISI. Minimum specimen size is 1 mL.

Important Precaution

GLP specimens must be collected using the GI Preservative tube. No other specimens are acceptable.

Special Specimens

For tumor/tissue and various fluids (e.g., CSF, peritoneal fluid, synovial fluid) contact ISI for requirements and special handling instructions.

Shipping Instructions

Specimens should be shipped frozen in dry ice.

References

1. Philippe J, Mojsov S, Drucker DJ, et al. Proglucagon processing in a rat islet cell line resembles phenotype of intestine rather than pancreas. Endocrinology. Dec;119(6):2833-9, 1986.
2. Weir GC, Mojsov S, Hendrick GK, et al. Glucagonlike peptide I (7-37) actions on endocrine pancreas. Diabetes. Mar;38(3):338-42, 1989.
3. Meier JJ, Nauck MA. Clinical endocrinology and metabolism. Glucose-dependent insulinotropic polypeptide/gastric inhibitory polypeptide. Best Pract Res Clin Endocrinol Metab. 18(4):587-606, 2004.
4. Nauck MA, Baller B, Meier JJ. Gastric inhibitory polypeptide and glucagon-like peptide-1 in the pathogenesis of type 2 diabetes. Diabetes. 53(Suppl 3):S190-6, 2004.
5. Drucker DJ. Glucagon-like peptides. Diabetes. 47(2):159-69, 1998.
6. Drucker DJ. Biological actions and therapeutic potential of the glucagon-like peptides. Gastroenterology. 122(2): 531-44, 2002.
7. Lovshin J, Drucker DJ. Synthesis, secretion and biological actions of the glucagon-like peptides. Pediatr Diabetes. 1(1):49-57, 2000.

CPT Code:
Unspecified Quantitative Immunoassay 83519

GROWTH HORMONE (GH, SOMATOTROPIN)

Reference Ranges

Children: up to 20 ng/mL
Adults: up to 10 ng/mL
Reference range is listed on individual patient test reports.

Procedure

GH is measured by direct radioimmunoassay.

Patient Preparation

The patient should not be on any insulin therapy nor take ACTH or gonadotropin medication, if possible, for at least 48 hours prior to collection of specimen.

Specimen Collection

Collect 3 mL serum or EDTA plasma and separate as soon as possible. Freeze plasma immediately after separation. Minimum specimen size is 1 mL.

Special Specimens

For tumor/tissue and various fluids (e.g., CSF, peritoneal fluid, synovial fluid) contact ISI for requirements and special handling instructions.

Shipping Instructions

Specimens should be shipped at room temperature or frozen in dry ice.

References

1. Word RA, Odom MJ, Byrd W, et al. The effect of gonadotropin-releasing hormone Agonists on growth hormone secretion in adult premenopausal women. Fertil Steril. Jul;54(1):73-8, 1990.
2. Strasburger C, Barnard G, Toldo L, et al. Somatotropin as measured by a two-site time-resolved immunofluorometric assay. Clin Chem. Jun;35(6):913-7, 1989.
3. Sheppard MC. Growth hormone—from molecule to mortality. Clin Med. 4(5):437-40, 2004.

CPT Code:
Growth Hormone 83003

GROWTH HORMONE–RELEASING HORMONE (GHRH)

Reference Range

5–18 pg/mL
Reference range is listed on individual patient test reports.

Procedure

GHRH is measured by direct radioimmunoassay.

Patient Preparation

The patient should not take any medications that influence pituitary secretion, if possible, for at least 48 hours prior to collection of specimen.

Specimen Collection

Collect 3 mL serum or EDTA plasma and separate as soon as possible. Freeze serum or plasma immediately after separation. Minimum specimen size is 1 mL.

Special Specimens

For tumor/tissue and various fluids (e.g., CSF, peritoneal fluid, synovial fluid) contact ISI for requirements and special handling instructions.

Shipping Instructions

Specimens should be shipped frozen in dry ice.

References

1. Vance ML. Growth-hormone releasing hormone. Clin Chem. 36:415-20, 1990.
2. Sopwith AM, Penny ES, Grossman A, et al. Normal circulating growth hormone releasing factor (hGRF) concentrations in patients with functional hypothalamic hGRF deficiency. Clin Endocrinol (Oxf). 24:395-400, 1986.
3. Groot K, Csernus VJ, Pinski J, et al. Development of a radioimmunoassay for some agonists of growth hormone-releasing hormone. Int J Pept Protein Res. 41(2):162-8, 1993.
4. DeLellis RA, Xia L. Paraneoplastic endocrine syndromes: a review. Endocr Pathol. 14(4):303-17, 2003.

CPT Code:
Growth Hormone–Releasing Hormone 83519

HISTAMINE

Reference Range

Up to 60 ng/mL
Reference range is listed on individual patient test reports.

Procedure

Histamine is measured by direct radioimmunoassay.

Patient Preparation

The patient should not take any antihistamine medication, if possible, for at least 48 hours prior to collection of specimen.

Specimen Collection

Collect 3 mL serum or EDTA plasma and separate as soon as possible. Freeze serum or plasma immediately after separation. Minimum specimen size is 1 mL.

Special Specimens

For tumor/tissue and various fluids (e.g., CSF, peritoneal fluid, synovial fluid), contact ISI for requirements and special handling instructions.

Shipping Instructions

Specimens should be shipped frozen in dry ice.

References

1. Marquardt DL. Histamine. Clin Rev Allergy. Sep;1(3):343-51, 1983.
2. Harsing LG Jr, Nagashima H, Duncalf D, et al. Determination of histamine concentrations in plasma by liquid chromatography/electrochemistry. Clin Chem (Oxf). Oct;32(10):1823-7, 1986.

CPT Code:
Histamine 83088

Homocysteine*

Reference Range

Reference range is listed on individual patient test reports.

Procedure

Homocysteine is measured by direct radioimmunoassay.

Patient Preparation

The patient should fast for 10 to 12 hours prior to collection of specimen. Antacid medications and medications that affect intestinal motility or insulin secretion should be discontinued, if possible, for at least 48 hours prior to collection of specimen.

Specimen Collection

Collect 10 mL EDTA plasma and separate as soon as possible. Freeze plasma immediately after separation. Minimum specimen size is 2 mL.

Shipping Instructions

Specimens should be shipped frozen in dry ice.

Reference

1. Please refer to www.endotext.org.

*** In preparation**

CPT Code:
Homocysteine 83090

Insulin

Reference Range

4–24 µU/mL
Reference range is listed on individual patient test reports.

Procedure

Insulin is measured by direct radioimmunoassay.

Patient Preparation

The patient should fast for 10 to 12 hours prior to collection of specimen. The patient should not take any medications that influence insulin production or secretion, if possible, for at least 48 hours prior to collection of specimen.

Specimen Collection

Collect 3 mL serum and separate as soon as possible. Freeze serum immediately after separation. Minimum specimen size is 1 mL.

Special Specimens

For tumor/tissue and various fluids (e.g., CSF, peritoneal fluid, synovial fluid) contact ISI for requirements and special handling instructions.

Shipping Instructions

Specimens should be shipped frozen in dry ice.

References

1. Wild RA, Applebaum-Bowden D, Demers LM, et alJ. Lipoprotein lipids in women with androgen excess: independent associations with increased insulin and androgen. Clin Chem (Oxf). 36:283-9, 1990.
2. Argoud GM, Schad DS, Eaton RP. Insulin suppresses its own secretion in vivo. Diabetes. 36:959-62, 1987.
3. Chevenne D, Trivin F, Porquet D. Insulin assays and reference values. Diabetes Metab. 25(6):459-76, 1999.

CPT Codes:

Insulin 80422,
80432–80435
- Antibody 86337
- Blood 83525
- Free 83527

Insulin, "Free"

Reference Range

4–24 μU/mL
Reference range is listed on individual patient test reports.

Procedure

"Free" insulin is measured by radioimmunoassay following removal of insulin bound to insulin antibodies.

Patient Preparation

The patient should fast for 10 to 12 hours prior to collection of specimen. The patient should not take any medications that influence insulin production or secretion, if possible, for at least 48 hours prior to collection of specimen.

Specimen Collection

Collect 3 mL serum or EDTA plasma and separate as soon as possible. Freeze serum or plasma immediately after separation. Minimum specimen size is 1 mL.

Shipping Instructions

Specimens should be shipped frozen in dry ice.

References

1. Hanning I, Home PD, Alberti KGMM. Measurement of free insulin concentrations: the influence of the timing of extraction of insulin antibodies. Diabetologia. 28:831-5, 1985.
2. Chevenne D, Valade F, Bridel MP, et al. Protein A-sepharose used to measure free insulin in plasma. Clin Chem (Oxf). 37:64-7, 1991.
3. Sapin R. Insulin assays: previously known and new analytical features. Clin Lab. 49(3-4):113-21, 2003

CPT Code:
"Free" Insulin 83527

INSULIN ANTIBODIES

Reference Range

Nondetectable
Reference range is listed on individual patient test reports.

Procedure

Insulin antibody determination is measured by radioimmunoassay.

Patient Preparation

The patient should fast for 10 to 12 hours prior to collection of specimen. Patients on insulin therapy with signs of insulin resistance are the most likely to test positive for insulin antibodies.

Specimen Collection

Collect 3 mL serum or EDTA plasma and separate as soon as possible. Freeze serum or plasma immediately after separation. Minimum specimen size is 1 mL.

Shipping Instructions

Specimens should be shipped frozen in dry ice.

References

1. Diaz JL, Wilkins TJ. Effect of iodination site on binding radiolabeled ligand by insulin antibodies and insulin autoantibodies. Clin Chem (Oxf). 34:356-9, 1988.
2. Patterson R, Mellies CJ, Roberts M. Immunologic reactions against insulin III. IgE anti¬insulin, insulin allergy, and combined IgE and IgG immuno¬logic insulin resistance. J Immunol. 110:1135, 1973.
3. Savola K, Sabbah E, Kulmala P, et al. Autoantibodies associated with type I diabetes mellitus persist after diagnosis in children. Diabetologia 41(11):1293-7, 1998.

CPT Code:
Insulin Antibody 86337

INSULIN—PROINSULIN

Reference Ranges

Proinsulin in normal fasting plasma is usually 10% to 15% and always less than 22% of total insulin.

Proinsulin component in fasting plasma of patients with islet cell disease is greater than 22% of total insulin.

Reference range is listed on individual patient test reports.

Procedure

Proinsulin is measured by radioimmunoassay following chromatographic purification of specimens.

Patient Preparation

The patient should fast for 10 to 12 hours prior to collection of specimen. The patient should not take any medications that influence insulin production or secretion, if possible, for at least 48 hours prior to collection of specimen.

Specimen Collection

Collect 3 mL serum or EDTA plasma and separate as soon as possible. Freeze serum or plasma immediately after separation. Minimum specimen size is 1 mL.

Special Specimens

For tumor/tissue and various fluids (e.g., CSF, peritoneal fluid, synovial fluid) contact ISI for requirements and special handling instructions.

Shipping Instructions

Specimens should be shipped frozen in dry ice.

References

1. Ward WK, Paquette TL, Frank BH, et al. A sensitive radioimmunoassay for human proinsulin with sequential use of antisera to peptide and insulin. Clin Chem (Oxf). 32:728-33, 1986.
2. Shetty MR, Boghossian HM, Duffell D, et al. Tumor-induced hypoglycemia: a result of ectopic insulin production. Cancer. 1 May;49(9):1920-3, 1982.
3. Rutter GA. Insulin secretion: feed-forward control of insulin biosynthesis? Curr Biol. 9(12):R443-4, 1999.
4. Sapin R. Insulin assays: previously known and new analytical features. Clin Lab. 49(3-4):113-21, 2003.
5. Jia EZ, Yang ZJ, Chen SW, Qi GY, You CF, Ma JF, Zhang JX, Wang ZZ, Qian WC, Li XL, Wang HY, Ma WZ. Significant association of insulin and proinsulin with clustering of cardiovascular risk factors. World J Gastroenterol. 11(1): 149-53, 2005.
6. Pfutzner A, Pfutzner AH, Larbig M, Forst T. Role of intact proinsulin in diagnosis and treatment of type 2 diabetes mellitus. Diabetes Technol Ther. 6(3):405-12, 2004.
7. Wiesli P, Perren A, Saremaslani P, Pfammatter T, Spinas GA, Schmid C. Abnormalities of proinsulin processing in functioning insulinomas: clinical implications. Clin Endocrinol (Oxf). 61(4):424-30, 2004.
8. Gama R, Teale JD, Marks V. Best practice No 173: clinical and laboratory investigation of adult spontaneous hypoglycaemia. J Clin Pathol. 56(9):641-6, 2003.
9. Pozzilli P, Manfrini S, Monetini L. Biochemical markers of type 1 diabetes: clinical use. Scand J Clin Lab Invest (Suppl). 235:38-44, 2001.

CPT Codes:
Proinsulin 84206
Proinsulin Serum 84206

Leptin*

Reference Range

Reference range is listed on individual patient test reports.

Procedure

Leptin is measured by direct radioimmunoassay.

Patient Preparation

The patient should fast for 10 to 12 hours prior to collection of specimen. The patient should not take any medications that influence insulin production or secretion, if possible.

Specimen Collection

Collect 3 mL serum or EDTA plasma and separate as soon as possible. Freeze serum or plasma immediately after separation. Minimum specimen size is 1 mL.

Special Specimens

For tumor/tissue and various fluids (e.g., CSF, peritoneal fluid, synovial fluid) contact ISI for requirements and special handling instructions.

Shipping Instructions

Specimens should be shipped frozen in dry ice.

References

1. Valle M, Martos R, Gascon F, et al. Low-grade systemic inflammation, hypoadiponectinemia and a high concentration of leptin are present in very young obese children, and correlate with metabolic syndrome. Diabetes Metab. Feb;31(1):55-62, 2005.
2. Er H, Doganay S, Ozerol E, et al. Adrenomedullin and leptin levels in diabetic retinopathy and retinal diseases. Ophthalmologica. Mar-Apr;219(2):107-11, 2005.
3. Mars M, de Graaf C, de Groot LC, et al. Decreases in fasting leptin and insulin concentrations after acute energy restriction and subsequent compensation in food intake. Am J Clin Nutr. Mar;81(3):570-7, 2005.
4. Abdella NA, Mojiminiyi OA, Moussa MA, Zaki M, Al Mohammedi H, Al Ozairi ES, Al Jebely S. Plasma leptin concentration in patients with Type 2 diabetes: relationship to cardiovascular disease risk factors and insulin resistance. Diabet Med. Mar;22(3):278-85, 2005.
5. Boden G, Sargrad K, Homko C, Mozzoli M, Stein TP. Effect of a low-carbohydrate diet on appetite, blood glucose levels, and insulin resistance in obese patients with type 2 diabetes. Ann Intern Med. 15 Mar;142(6):403-11, 2005.

*** In preparation**

CPT Code:
Unspecified Quantitative Immunoassay 83519

Motilin

Reference Range

Up to 446 pg/mL
Reference range is listed on individual patient test reports.

Procedure

Motilin is measured by direct radioimmunoassay.

Patient Preparation

The patient should fast for 10 to 12 hours prior to collection of specimen. Antacid medications and medications that affect intestinal motility should be discontinued, if possible, for at least 48 hours prior to collection of specimen.

Specimen Collection

Collect 3 mL serum or EDTA plasma and separate as soon as possible. Freeze serum or plasma immediately after separation. Minimum specimen size is 1 mL.

Special Specimens

For tumor/tissue and various fluids (e.g., CSF, peritoneal fluid, synovial fluid) contact ISI for requirements and special handling instructions.

Shipping Instructions

Specimens should be shipped at room temperature or frozen in dry ice.

References

1. Dea D, Boileau G, Poitras P, et al. Molecular heterogeneity of human motilin like immunoreactivity explained by the processing of prepromotilin. Gastroenterology. Mar;96(3):695-703.
2. Vantrappen G, Janssens J, Peeters TL, et al. Motilin and the interdigestive migrating motor complex in man. Dig Dis Sci. Jul;24(7):497-500, 1979.
3. Vazeou A, Papadopoulou A, Papadimitriou A, et al. Autonomic neuropathy and gastrointestinal motility disorders in children and adolescents with type 1 diabetes mellitus. J Pediatr Gastroenterol Nutr. 38(1):61-5, 2004.
4. Ishikawa M, Raskin P. From motilin to motilides: a new direction in gastrointestinal endocrinology. Endocr Pract. 1(3):179-84, 1995.
5. Asakawa A, Inui A, Kaga T, et al. Ghrelin is an appetite-stimulatory signal from stomach with structural resemblance to motilin. Gastroenterology. 120(2):337-45, 2001.
6. Kamerling IM, Van Haarst AD, Burggraaf J, et al. Motilin effects on the proximal stomach in patients with functional dyspepsia and healthy volunteers. Am J Physiol Gastrointest Liver Physiol. 284(5):G776-81, 2003.
7. De Giorgio R, Barbara G, Stanghellini V, et al. Review article: the pharmacological treatment of acute colonic pseudo-obstruction. Aliment Pharmacol Ther. 15(11):1717-27, 2001.
8. Fiasse R, Deprez P, Weynand B, et al. An unusual metastatic motilin-secreting neuroendocrine tumour with a 20-year survival. Pathological, biochemical and motility features. Digestion. 64(4):255-60, 2001.

CPT Code:
Unspecified Quantitative Immunoassay 83519

NEUROKININ A (NKA; SUBSTANCE K)

Reference Range

Up to 40 pg/mL
Reference range is listed on individual patient test reports.

Procedure

NKA is measured by direct radioimmunoassay.

Patient Preparation

The patient should not take pain relievers or any medications that affect hypertension or gastrointestinal functions, if possible, for at least 48 hours prior to collection of specimen.

Specimen Collection

Collect 10 mL EDTA plasma in special tube containing the Z-tube™ Preservative and separate as soon as possible. Freeze plasma immediately after separation. Special Z-tube™ Preservative is available from ISI. Minimum specimen size is 1 mL.

Special Specimens

For tumor/tissue and various fluids (e.g., CSF, peritoneal fluid, synovial fluid) contact ISI for requirements and special handling instructions.

Shipping Instructions

Specimens should be shipped frozen in dry ice.

References

1. Kimuro S, Okada M, Sugata Y. Novel neuropeptides neurokinin alpha and beta, isolated from porcine spinal cord. Proc Japan Acad. 59:101, 1983.
2. Nawa H, Kotani H, Nakanishi S. Tissue specific generation of tissue pre-pro-tachykinin mRNAs from one gene by alternative RNA splicing. Nature. 20 Dec-2 Jan 2;312(5996):729-34, 1984-5.
3. Theodorsson-Norheim E, Norheim I, et alG. Neuropeptide K: a major tachykinin in plasma and tumor tissues from carcinoid patients. Biochem Biophys Res Commun. 131(1):77-83, 1985.
4. Conlon JM, Deacon CF, Richter G, et al. Measurement and partial characterization of the multiple forms of neurokinin A-like immunoreactivity in carcinoid tumours. Regul Pept. Jan;13(2):183-96, 1986.
5. Hunt RH, Tougas G. Evolving concepts in functional gastrointestinal disorders: promising directions for novel pharmaceutical treatments. Best Pract Res Clin Gastroenterol. 16(6):869-83, 2002.
6. Ardill JE, Erikkson B. The importance of the measurement of circulating markers in patients with neuroendocrine tumours of the pancreas and gut. Endocr Relat Cancer. 10(4):459-62, 2003.
7. Chen LW, Yung KK, Chan YS. Neurokinin peptides and neurokinin receptors as potential therapeutic intervention targets of basal ganglia in the prevention and treatment of Parkinson's disease. Curr Drug Targets. 5(2):197-206, 2004.
8. Severini C, Ciotti MT, Mercanti D, et al. The tachykinin peptide family. Pharmacol Rev. 54(2):285-322, 2002.
9. Pennefather JN, Lecci A, Candenas ML, et al. Tachykinins and tachykinin receptors: a growing family. Life Sci. 74(12):1445-63, 2004.

CPT Code:
Unspecified Quantitative Immunoassay 83519

NEUROPEPTIDE Y (NPY)

Reference Range

Up to 5.0 ng/mL
Reference range is listed on individual patient test reports.

Procedure

NPY is measured by direct radioimmunoassay.

Patient Preparation

The patient should fast for 10 to 12 hours prior to collection of specimen. Medications that affect insulin secretion or gastrointestinal function should be discontinued, if possible, for at least 48 hours prior to collection of specimen.

Specimen Collection

Collect 3 mL serum or EDTA plasma and separate as soon as possible. Freeze serum or plasma immediately after separation. Minimum specimen size is 1 mL.

Special Specimens

For tumor/tissue and various fluids (e.g., CSF, peritoneal fluid, synovial fluid) contact ISI for requirements and special handling instructions.

Shipping Instructions

Specimens should be shipped frozen in dry ice.

References

1. Jamal H, Jones PM, Byrne J, et al. Peptide contents of neuropeptide Y, vasoactive intestinal polypeptide, and β-calcitonin gene-related peptide and their messenger ribonucleic acids after dexamethasone treatment in the isolated rat islets of langerhans. Endocrinology. 129:3372-80, 1991.
2. Lehmann J. Neuropeptide Y: an overview. Drug Dev Res. 19:329-51, 1989.
3. O'Dorisio MS, Hauger M, O'Dorisio TM. Age-dependent levels of plasma neuropeptides in normal children. Regul Pept. 109(1-3):189-92, 2002.
4. Gehlert DR. Introduction to the reviews on neuropeptide Y. Neuropeptides. 38(4):135-40, 2004.
5. Zoccali C. Neuropeptide Y as a far-reaching neuromediator: from energy balance and cardiovascular regulation to central integration of weight and bone mass control mechanisms. Implications for human diseases. Curr Opin Nephrol Hypertens. 14(1):25-32, 2005.
6. Beaujouan JC, Torrens Y, Saffroy M, et al. A 25 year adventure in the field of tachykinins. Peptides. 25(3):339-57, 2004.
7. Oberg K. Biochemical diagnosis of neuroendocrine GEP tumor. Yale J Biol Med. 70(5-6):501-8, 1997.
8. Makridis C, Theodorsson E, Akerstrom G, et al. Increased intestinal non-substance P tachykinin concentrations in malignant midgut carcinoid disease. J Gastroenterol Hepatol. 14(5):500-7, 1999.

CPT Code:
Unspecified Quantitative Immunoassay 83519

Neurotensin

Reference Range

50–100 pg/mL
Reference range is listed on individual patient test reports.

Procedure

Neurotensin is measured by direct radioimmunoassay.

Patient Preparation

The patient should fast for 10 to 12 hours prior to collection of specimen. Antacid medications and medications that affect gastrointestinal function should be discontinued, if possible, for at least 48 hours prior to collection of specimen.

Specimen Collection

Collect 10 mL EDTA plasma in special tube containing the Z-tube™ Preservative and separate as soon as possible. Freeze plasma immediately after separation. Special Z-tube™ Preservative is available from ISI. Minimum specimen size is 1 mL.

Special Specimens

For tumor/tissue and various fluids (e.g., CSF, peritoneal fluid, synovial fluid) contact ISI for requirements and special handling instructions.

Shipping Instructions

Specimens should be shipped frozen in dry ice.

References

1. Shulkes A, Chick P, Wong H, et al. A radioimmunoassay for neurotensin in human plasma. Clin Chim Acta. 13 Oct;125(1):49-58, 1982.
2. Carraway RE, Mitra SP, Feurle GE, et al. Presence of neurotensin and neuromedin-N within a common precursor from a human pancreatic neuroendocrine tumor. J Clin Endocrinol Metab. Jun;66(6):1323-8. 1988.
3. Reubi JC. Peptide receptors as molecular targets for cancer diagnosis and therapy. Endocr Rev. 24(4):389-427, 2003.

CPT Code:
Unspecified Quantitative Immunoassay 83519

NUCLEAR FACTOR KAPPA B (NFκB)*

Reference Range

Reference range is listed on individual patient test reports.

Procedure

NFκB is measured by direct radioimmunoassay.

Patient Preparation

The patient should fast for 10 to 12 hours prior to collection of specimen. The patient should not take any medications that influence insulin production or secretion, if possible, for at least 48 hours prior to collection of specimen.

Specimen Collection

Collect 3 mL serum or EDTA plasma and separate as soon as possible. Freeze serum or plasma immediately after separation. Minimum specimen size is 1 mL.

Special Specimens

For tumor/tissue and various fluids (e.g., CSF, peritoneal fluid, synovial fluid) contact ISI for requirements and special handling instructions.

Shipping Instructions

Specimens should be shipped frozen in dry ice.

Reference

1. Dhindsa S, Tripathy D, Mohanty P, et al. Differential effects of glucose and alcohol on reactive oxygen species generation and intranuclear nuclear factor-kappa B in mononuclear cells. Metabolism. Mar;53(3):330-4, 2004.

*** In preparation**

CPT Code:
Unspecified Quantitative Immunoassay 83519

OCTREOTIDE (SANDOSTATIN®)

Reference Ranges for Therapeutic Octreotide Levels

Long-acting repeatable (LAR) dose-response levels: mean octreotide level ± 2 SD for patients on octreotide LAR for 3 or more months (steady-state). The following represent trough levels measured immediately before an injection of LAR.

10 mg/month: 1,153 ± 748 pg/mL
20 mg/month: 2,518 ± 1,020 pg/mL
30 mg/month: 5,241 ± 3,004 pg/mL
60 mg/month: 10,926 ± 5,530 pg/mL

Procedure

Octreotide is measured by direct radioimmunoassay. There is no cross-reactivity with native somatostatin-14 or somatostatin-28. The also is no cross-reactivity with lanreotide, and this test should not be used to measure blood levels of this drug.

Patient Preparation

This test is useful only for those patients being treated with octreotide acetate. No special preparation is needed for this test. For optimal results, blood for this test should be drawn immediately before the patient's next injection of octreotide LAR (trough levels).

Specimen Collection

Collect 3 mL serum or EDTA plasma and separate as soon as possible. Octreotide is stable at room temperature for 3 days. Specimens can be stored at room temperature, refrigerated, or frozen in dry ice. Minimum specimen size is 1 mL.

Special Specimens

For tumor/tissue and various fluids (e.g., CSF, peritoneal fluid, synovial fluid) contact ISI for requirements and special handling instructions.

Shipping Instructions

Specimens can be shipped at ambient temperature, refrigerated, or frozen in dry ice.

Reference

1. Woltering EA, Mamikunian PM, Zietz S, et al. The effect of octreotide LAR dose and weight on octreotide blood levels in patients with neuroendocrine tumors. Pancreas. 31(4):392-400, 2005.

CPT Code:
Therapeutic Drug Assay: Quantitation of Drug, Not Elsewhere Specified 80299

PANCREASTATIN

Reference Range

10–135 pg/mL
Reference range is listed on individual patient test reports.

Procedure

Pancreastatin is measured by direct radioimmunoassay/EIA/ELISA.

Patient Preparation

The patient should fast for 10 to 12 hours prior to collection of specimen. The patient should not take any medications that influence insulin levels, if possible, for at least 48 hours prior to collection of specimen.

Specimen Collection

Collect 10 mL EDTA plasma in special tube containing the Z-tube™ Preservative and separate as soon as possible. Freeze plasma immediately after separation. Special Z-tube™ Preservative is available from ISI. Minimum specimen size is 1 mL.

Special Specimens

For tumor/tissue and various fluids (e.g., CSF, peritoneal fluid, synovial fluid) contact ISI for requirements and special handling instructions.

Shipping Instructions

Specimens should be shipped frozen in dry ice.

References

1. Piero E, Mirelles P, Silvestre RA, et al. Pancreastatin inhibits insulin secretion as induced by glucagon, vasoactive intestinal polypeptide, gastric inhibiting peptide, and 8-cholecystokinin in the perfused rat pancreas. Metabolism. 38:679-82, 1989.
2. Tatemoto K, Efendi S, Mutt S, et al. Pancreastatin, a novel pancreatic peptide that inhibits insulin secretion. Nature. 324:476-8, 1986.
3. Calhoun K, Toth-Fejel S, Chee J, et al. Serum peptide profiles in patients with carcinoid tumors. Am J Surg. 186(1): 28-31, 2003.
4. Syversen U, Jacobsen MB, O'Connor DT, et al. Immunoassays for measurement of chromogranin A and pancreastatin-like immunoreactivity in humans: correspondence in patients with neuroendocrine neoplasia. Neuropeptides. 26(3):201-6, 1994.
5. Kogner P, Bjellerup P, Svensson T, et al. Pancreastatin immunoreactivity in favourable childhood neuroblastoma and ganglioneuroma. Eur J Cancer 31A(4):557-60, 1995.
6. Desai DC, O'Dorisio TM, Schirmer WJ, et al. Serum pancreastatin levels predict response to hepatic artery chemoembolization and somatostatin analogue therapy in metastatic neuroendocrine tumors. Regul Pept. 96(3):113-17, 2001.

CPT Code:
Unspecified Quantitative Immunoassay 83519

PANCREATIC POLYPEPTIDE (PP)

Reference Ranges

Age (y)	Range (pg/mL)
20–29	10–140
30–39	20–500
40–49	25–880
50–59	25–925
60–69	40–600

Reference range is listed on individual patient test reports.

Procedure

PP is measured by direct radioimmunoassay.

Patient Preparation

The patient should fast for 10 to 12 hours prior to collection of specimen. Antacid medications and medications that affect insulin levels should be discontinued, if possible, for at least 48 hours prior to collection of specimen.

Specimen Collection

Collect 3 mL serum or EDTA plasma and separate as soon as possible. Freeze serum or plasma immediately after separation. Minimum specimen size is 1 mL.

Special Specimens

For tumor/tissue and various fluids (e.g., CSF, peritoneal fluid, synovial fluid) contact ISI for requirements and special handling instructions.

Shipping Instructions

Specimens should be shipped frozen in dry ice.

References

1. Kennedy FP, Go VLW, Cryer PE, et al. Subnormal pancreatic polypeptide and epinephrine response to insulin-induced hypoglycemia identify patients with insulin-dependent diabetes mellitus predisposal to develop overt autonomic neuropathy. Ann Intern Med. Jan;108(1):54-8, 1988.
2. Stern AI, Hansky J. Pancreatic polypeptide release in gastric ulcer. Dig Dis Sci. Apr;26(4):289-91, 1981.
3. Druce MR, Small CJ, Bloom SR. Minireview: gut peptides regulating satiety. Endocrinology. 145(6):2660-5, 2004.
4. Small CJ, Bloom SR. Gut hormones and the control of appetite. Trends Endocrinol Metab. 15(6):259-63, 2004.
5. Batterham RL, Le Roux CW, Cohen MA, et al. Pancreatic polypeptide reduces appetite and food intake in humans. J Clin Endocrinol Metab. 88(8):3989-92, 2003.
6. Panzuto F, Severi C, Cannizzaro R, et al. Utility of combined use of plasma levels of chromogranin A and pancreatic polypeptide in the diagnosis of gastrointestinal and pancreatic endocrine tumors. J Endocrinol Invest. 27(1):6-11, 2004.
7. Yamashita Y, Miyahara E, Shimizu K, et al. Screening of gastrointestinal hormone release in patients with lung cancer. In Vivo. 17(2):193-5, 2003.

CPT Code:
Unspecified Quantitative Immunoassay 83519

PEPSINOGEN I (PG-I)

Reference Range

28–100 ng/mL
Reference range is listed on individual patient test reports.

Procedure

PG-I is measured by direct radioimmunoassay.

Patient Preparation

The patient should fast for 10 to 12 hours prior to collection of specimen. Antacid medications or medications that affect intestinal motility should be discontinued, if possible, for at least 48 hours prior to collection of specimen.

Specimen Collection

Collect 3 mL serum or EDTA plasma and separate as soon as possible. Freeze serum or plasma immediately after separation. Minimum specimen size is 1 mL.

Special Specimens

For tumor/tissue and various fluids (e.g., CSF, peritoneal fluid, synovial fluid) contact ISI for requirements and special handling instructions.

Shipping Instructions

Specimens should be shipped frozen in dry ice.

References

1. Plebani M, DiMario F, Dal Santo PL, et al. Measurement of pepsinogen group I in endoscopic gastroduodenal biopsies. Clin Chem. 36:682-4, 1990.
2. Samloff IM, Liebman WM. Radioimmunoassay of group I pepsinogens in serum. Gastroenterology. Apr;66(4): 494-502, 1974.

CPT Code:
Unspecified Quantitative Immunoassay 83519

PEPSINOGEN II (PG-II)

Reference Range

Up to 22 ng/mL
Reference range is listed on individual patient test reports.

Procedure

PG-II is measured by direct radioimmunoassay.

Patient Preparation

The patient should fast for 10 to 12 hours prior to collection of specimen. Antacid medications or medications that affect intestinal motility should be discontinued, if possible, for at least 48 hours prior to collection of specimen.

Specimen Collection

Collect 3 mL serum or EDTA plasma and separate as soon as possible. Freeze serum or plasma immediately after separation. Minimum specimen size is 1 mL.

Special Specimens

For tumor/tissue and various fluids (e.g., CSF, peritoneal fluid, synovial fluid) contact ISI for requirements and special handling instructions.

Shipping Instructions

Specimens should be shipped frozen in dry ice.

References

1. Plebani M, Masiero M, DiMario F, et al. Radioimmunoassay for pepsinogen C. Clin Chem. Sep;36(9):1690, 1990.
2. Matzku S, Zoller M, Rapp W. Radioimmunological quantification of human group-II pepsinogens. Digestion. 18(1-2):16-26, 1978.

CPT Code:
Unspecified Quantitative Immunoassay 83519

Peptide Histidine Isoleucine (PHIM)*

Reference Range

10–40 pg/mL
Reference range is listed on individual patient test reports.

Procedure

PHIM is measured by direct radioimmunoassay.

Patient Preparation

The patient should fast for 10 to 12 hours prior to collection of specimen. Antacid medications and medications that affect intestinal motility should be discontinued, if possible, for at least 48 hours prior to collection of specimen.

Specimen Collection

Collect 10 mL EDTA plasma in a special tube containing the GI Preservative and separate as soon as possible. Freeze plasma immediately after separation. Special GI Preservative tubes are available from ISI. Minimum specimen size is 1 mL.

Important Precaution

PHIM specimens must be collected using the GI Preservative tube. No other specimens are acceptable.

Special Specimens

For tumor/tissue and various fluids (e.g., CSF, peritoneal fluid, synovial fluid) contact ISI for requirements and special handling instructions.

Shipping Instructions

Specimens should be shipped frozen in dry ice.

References

1. Yiango Y, Christofides ND, Blank MA, et al. Molecular forms of peptide histidine isoleucine-like immunoreactivity in the gastrointestinal tract. Gastroenterology. Sep;89(3):516-24, 1985.
2. Christofides ND, Yiangou Y, Aarons E. Radioimmunoassay and intramural distribution of PHI-IR in the human intestine. Dig Dis Sci. Jun;28(6):507-12, 1983.
3. Fahrenkrug J, Hannibal J. Neurotransmitters co-existing with VIP or PACAP. Peptides. 25(3):393-401, 2004.
4. D'Souza M, Plevak D, Kvols L, Shine T, Stapelfeldt W, Nelson D, Southorn P, Murray M. Elevated neuropeptide levels decrease during liver transplant. Transplant Proc. 25(2):1805-6, 1993.

*** In preparation**

CPT Code:
Unspecified Quantitative Immunoassay 83519

Peptide YY (PYY)

Reference Range

30–120 pg/mL
Reference range is listed on individual patient test reports.

Procedure

PYY is measured by direct radioimmunoassay.

Patient Preparation

The patient should fast for 10 to 12 hours prior to collection of specimen. Antacid medications and medications that affect intestinal motility should be discontinued, if possible, for at least 48 hours prior to collection of specimen.

Specimen Collection

Collect 10 mL EDTA plasma in a special tube containing the GI Preservative and separate as soon as possible. Freeze plasma immediately after separation. Special GI Preservative tubes are available from ISI. Minimum specimen size is 1 mL.

Important Precaution

PYY specimens must be collected using the GI Preservative tube. No other specimens are acceptable.

Special Specimens

For tumor/tissue and various fluids (e.g., CSF, peritoneal fluid, synovial fluid) contact ISI for requirements and special handling instructions.

Shipping Instructions

Specimens should be shipped frozen in dry ice.

References

1. Adrian TE, Ferri GL, Bacarese-Hamilton AJ, et al. Human distribution and release of a putative new gut hormone, peptide YY. Gastroenterology. Nov;89(5):1070-7, 1985.
2. Adrian TE, Bacarese-Hamilton AJ, Savage AP, et al. Peptide YY abnormalities in gastrointestinal diseases. Gastroenterology. Feb;90(2):379-84, 1986.
3. Lin HC, Chey WY. Cholecystokinin and peptide YY are released by fat in either proximal or distal small intestine in dogs. Regul Pept. 114(2-3):131-5, 2003.
4. McGowan BM, Bloom SR. Peptide YY and appetite control. Curr Opin Pharmacol. 4(6):583-8, 2004.

CPT Code:
Unspecified Quantitative Immunoassay 83519

PLASMINOGEN ACTIVATOR INHIBITOR 1 (PAI-1)*

Reference Range

Up to 1.0 IU/mL
Reference range is listed on individual patient test reports.

Procedure

PAI-1 is measured by direct radioimmunoassay.

Patient Preparation

The patient should fast for 10 to 12 hours prior to collection of specimen. Antacid medications and medications that affect intestinal motility should be discontinued, if possible, for at least 48 hours prior to collection of specimen.

Specimen Collection

Collect 10 mL EDTA plasma in a special tube containing the GI Preservative and separate as soon as possible. Freeze plasma immediately after separation. Special GI Preservative tubes are available from ISI. Minimum specimen size is 1 mL.

Important Precaution

PAI-1 specimens must be collected using the GI Preservative tube. No other specimens are acceptable.

Special Specimens

For tumor/tissue and various fluids (e.g., CSF, peritoneal fluid, synovial fluid) contact ISI for requirements and special handling instructions.

Shipping Instructions

Specimens should be shipped frozen in dry ice.

References

1. Juhan-Vague I, Alessi MC, Vague P. Increased plasma plasminogen activator inhibitor I levels. A possible link between insulin resistance and atherothrombosis. Diabetologia. 34:457-62, 1991.
2. Landin K, Tengborn L, Smith U. Elevated fibrinogen and plasminogen activator inhibitor (PAI-I) in hypertension are related to metabolic risk factors for cardiovascular disease. J Intern Med. 227:273-8, 1990.

*** In preparation**

CPT Codes:
PAI-1 85420–85421

PROSTAGLANDIN D_2 (PGD_2)

Reference Range

35–115 pg/mL
Reference range is listed on individual patient test reports.

Procedure

PGD_2 is measured by radioimmunoassay/EIA/ELISA following extraction of specimens.

Patient Preparation

The patient should not take aspirin, indomethacin, or anti-inflammatory medications, if possible, for at least 48 hours prior to collection of specimen.

Specimen Collection

Collect 3 mL serum or EDTA plasma and separate as soon as possible. Freeze serum or plasma immediately after separation. Minimum specimen size is 1 mL.

Special Specimens

For tumor/tissue and various fluids (e.g., CSF, peritoneal fluid, synovial fluid) contact ISI for requirements and special handling instructions.

Shipping Instructions

Specimens should be shipped frozen in dry ice.

References

1. Redfern JS, Feldman M. Role of endogenous prostaglandins in preventing gastrointestinal ulceration: induction of ulcers by antibodies to prostaglandins. Gastroenterology. Feb;96(2 Pt 2 Suppl):596-605, 1989.
2. Bennegard B, Hahlin M, Hamberger L. Luteotropic effects of prostaglandins I_2 and D_2 on isolated human corpora luteum. Fertil Steril. Sep;54(3):459-64, 1990.

CPT Code:
Prostaglandin D_2 84150

Prostaglandin D_2 (PGD_2), Urine

Reference Range

100–280 ng/24 hours
Reference range is listed on individual patient test reports.

Procedure

PGD_2 is measured by direct radioimmunoassay/EIA/ELISA.

Patient Preparation

The patient should not take aspirin, indomethacin, or anti-inflammatory medications, if possible, for at least 48 hours prior to collection of specimen.

Specimen Collection

Submit 5 mL of a 24-hour urine collection. No special preservatives are required. Minimum specimen size is 1 mL. Provide the total volume per 24 hours, if possible; random collections are also acceptable.

Shipping Instructions

Specimens should be shipped frozen in dry ice.

References

1. Redfern JS, Feldman M. Role of endogenous prostaglandins in preventing gastrointestinal ulceration: induction of ulcers by antibodies to prostaglandins. Gastroenterology. Feb;96(2 Pt 2 Suppl):596-605, 1989.
2. Bennegard B, Hahlin M, Hamberger L. Luteotropic effects of prostaglandins I_2 and D_2 on isolated human corpora luteum. Fertil Steril. Sep;54(3):459-64, 1990.

CPT Code:
Prostaglandin D_2 84150

PROSTAGLANDIN E_1 (PGE_1)

Reference Range

250–500 pg/mL
Reference range is listed on individual patient test reports.

Procedure

PGE_1 is measured by radioimmunoassay/EIA/ELISA following extraction of specimens.

Patient Preparation

The patient should not take aspirin, indomethacin, or anti-inflammatory medications, if possible, for at least 48 hours prior to collection of specimen.

Specimen Collection

Collect 3 mL serum or EDTA plasma and separate as soon as possible. Freeze serum or plasma immediately after separation. Minimum specimen size is 1 mL.

Special Specimens

For tumor/tissue and various fluids (e.g., CSF, peritoneal fluid, synovial fluid) contact ISI for requirements and special handling instructions.

Shipping Instructions

Specimens should be shipped frozen in dry ice.

References

1. Redfern JS, Feldman M. Role of endogenous prostaglandins in preventing gastrointestinal ulceration: induction of ulcers by antibodies to prostaglandins. Gastroenterology. Feb;96(2 Pt 2 Suppl):596-605, 1989.
2. Dunn MJ, Zambraski EJ. Renal effects of drugs that inhibit prostaglandin synthesis. Kidney Int. Nov;18(5):609-22, 1980.

CPT Code:
Prostaglandin E_1 84150

PROSTAGLANDIN E_2 (PGE_2)

Reference Range

250–400 pg/mL
Reference range is listed on individual patient test reports.

Procedure

PGE_2 is measured by radioimmunoassay/EIA/ELISA following extraction of specimens.

Patient Preparation

The patient should not take aspirin, indomethacin, or anti-inflammatory medications, if possible, for at least 48 hours prior to collection of specimen.

Specimen Collection

Collect 3 mL serum or EDTA plasma and separate as soon as possible. Freeze serum or plasma immediately after separation. Minimum specimen size is 1 mL.

Special Specimens

For tumor/tissue and various fluids (e.g., CSF, peritoneal fluid, synovial fluid) contact ISI for requirements and special handling instructions.

Shipping Instructions

Specimens should be shipped frozen in dry ice.

References

1. Redfern JS, Feldman M. Role of endogenous prostaglandins in preventing gastrointestinal ulceration: induction of ulcers by antibodies to prostaglandins. Gastroenterology. Feb;96(2 Pt 2 Suppl):596-605, 1989.
2. Balasch J, Arroyo V, Carmona F, et al. Severe ovarian hyperstimulation syndrome: role of peripheral vasodilation. Fertil Steril. Dec;56(6):1077-83, 1991.

CPT Code:
Prostaglandin E_2 84150

Prostaglandin E_2 Dihydroketo (DHK-PGE_2)

Reference Range

Up to 40 pg/mL
Reference range is listed on individual patient test reports.

Procedure

DHK-PGE_2 is measured by radioimmunoassay/EIA/ELISA y following extraction of specimens.

Patient Preparation

The patient should not take aspirin, indomethacin, or anti-inflammatory medications, if possible, for at least 48 hours prior to collection of specimen.

Specimen Collection

Collect 3 mL serum or EDTA plasma and separate as soon as possible. Freeze serum or plasma immediately after separation. Minimum specimen size is 1 mL.

Special Specimens

For tumor/tissue and various fluids (e.g., CSF, peritoneal fluid, synovial fluid) contact ISI for requirements and special handling instructions.

Shipping Instructions

Specimens should be shipped frozen in dry ice.

References

1. Redfern JS, Feldman M. Role of endogenous prostaglandins in preventing gastrointestinal ulceration: induction of ulcers by antibodies to prostaglandins. Gastroenterology. Feb;96(2 Pt 2 Suppl):596-605, 1989.
2. Samuelsson B, Green K. Endogenous levels of 15-keto-dihydro-prostaglandins in human plasma. Biochem Med. Nov;11(3):298-303, 1974.

CPT Code:
Prostaglandin E_2 84150

PROSTAGLANDIN $F_1\alpha$ ($PGF_1\alpha$)

Reference Range

30–100 pg/mL
Reference range is listed on individual patient test reports.

Procedure

$PGF_1\alpha$ is measured by radioimmunoassay/EIA/ELISA following extraction of specimens.

Patient Preparation

The patient should not take aspirin, indomethacin, or anti-inflammatory medications, if possible, for at least 48 hours prior to collection of specimen.

Specimen Collection

Collect 3 mL serum or EDTA plasma and separate as soon as possible. Freeze serum or plasma immediately after separation. Minimum specimen size is 1 mL.

Special Specimens

For tumor/tissue and various fluids (e.g., CSF, peritoneal fluid, synovial fluid) contact ISI for requirements and special handling instructions.

Shipping Instructions

Specimens should be shipped frozen in dry ice.

References

1. Redfern JS, Feldman M. Role of endogenous prostaglandins in preventing gastrointestinal ulceration: induction of ulcers by antibodies to prostaglandins. Gastroenterology. Feb;96(2 Pt 2 Suppl):596-605, 1989.
2. Dray F, Charbonnel B, Maclouf J. Radioimmunoassay of prostaglandins F alpha, E_1, and E_2 in human plasma. Eur J Clin Invest. 29 Jul;5(4):311-8, 1975.

CPT Code:
Prostaglandin $F_1\alpha$ 84150

PROSTAGLANDIN $F_1\alpha$ ($PGF_1\alpha$), URINE

Reference Range

50–400 ng/24 hours
Reference range is listed on individual patient test reports.

Procedure

$PGF_1\alpha$ is measured by direct radioimmunoassay/EIA/ELISA.

Patient Preparation

The patient should not take aspirin, indomethacin, or anti-inflammatory medications, if possible, for at least 48 hours prior to collection of specimen.

Specimen Collection

Submit 5 mL of a 24-hour urine collection. No special preservatives are required. Minimum specimen size is 1 mL. Provide the total volume of urine per 24 hours, if possible; random collections are also acceptable.

Shipping Instructions

Specimens should be shipped frozen in dry ice.

References

1. Redfern JS, Feldman M. Role of endogenous prostaglandins in preventing gastrointestinal ulceration: induction of ulcers by antibodies to prostaglandins. Gastroenterology. Feb;96(2 Pt 2 Suppl):596-605, 1989.
2. Dray F, Charbonnel B, Maclouf J. Radioimmunoassay of prostaglandins F alpha, E_1, and E_2 in human plasma. Eur J Clin Invest. 29 Jul;5(4):311-8, 1975.

CPT Code:
Prostaglandin $F_1\alpha$ 84150

PROSTAGLANDIN $F_1\alpha$, 6-KETO (6-KETO $PGF_1\alpha$), PROSTAGLANDIN I_2 (PGI_2) METABOLITE

Reference Range

Up to 15 pg/mL
Reference range is listed on individual patient test reports.

Procedure

6-Keto $PGF_1\alpha$ is measured by radioimmunoassay/EIA/ELISA following extraction of specimens.

Patient Preparation

The patient should not take aspirin, indomethacin, or anti-inflammatory medications, if possible, for at least 48 hours prior to collection of specimen.

Specimen Collection

Collect 3 mL serum or EDTA plasma and separate as soon as possible. Freeze serum or plasma immediately after separation. Minimum specimen size is 1 mL.

Special Specimens

For tumor/tissue and various fluids (e.g., CSF, peritoneal fluid, synovial fluid) contact ISI for requirements and special handling instructions.

Shipping Instructions

Specimens should be shipped frozen in dry ice.

References

1. Redfern JS, Feldman M. Role of endogenous prostaglandins in preventing gastrointestinal ulceration: induction of ulcers by antibodies to prostaglandins. Gastroenterology. Feb;96(2 Pt 2 Suppl):596-605, 1989.
2. Schramm W, Smith RH, Jackson TM, et al. Rapid solid-phase immunoassay for 6-keto prostaglandin $F_1\alpha$ on microplates. Clin Chem. 36:509-14, 1990.

CPT Code:
Prostaglandin $F_1\alpha$ 84150

PROSTAGLANDIN $F_1\alpha$, 6-KETO (6-KETO $PGF_1\alpha$), PGI_2 METABOLITE, URINE

Reference Ranges

Male: 200–450 ng/24 hours
Female: 85–300 ng/24 hours
Reference range is listed on individual patient test reports.

Procedure

6-Keto $PGF_1\alpha$ is measured by direct radioimmunoassay/EIA/ELISA.

Patient Preparation

The patient should not take aspirin, indomethacin, or anti-inflammatory medications, if possible, for at least 48 hours prior to collection of specimen.

Specimen Collection

Submit 5 mL of a 24-hour urine collection. No special preservatives are required. Minimum specimen size is 1 mL. Provide total volume per 24 hours, if possible; random collections are also acceptable.

Shipping Instructions

Specimens should be shipped frozen in dry ice.

References

1. Redfern JS, Feldman M. Role of endogenous prostaglandins in preventing gastrointestinal ulceration: induction of ulcers by antibodies to prostaglandins. Gastroenterology. Feb;96(2 Pt 2 Suppl):596-605, 1989.
2. Zureick S, Nadler J, Yamamoto J, et al. Simultaneous measurement of two major prostacyclin metabolites in urine. Clin Chem. Nov;36(11):1978-80, 1990.

CPT Code:
Prostaglandin $F_1\alpha$ 84150

PROSTAGLANDIN $F_2\alpha$ ($PGF_2\alpha$)

Reference Range

80–240 pg/mL
Reference range is listed on individual patient test reports.

Procedure

$PGF_2\alpha$ is measured by radioimmunoassay/EIA/ELISA following extraction of specimens.

Patient Preparation

The patient should not take aspirin, indomethacin, or anti-inflammatory medications, if possible, for at least 48 hours prior to collection of specimen.

Specimen Collection

Collect 3 mL serum or EDTA plasma and separate as soon as possible. Freeze serum or plasma immediately after separation. Minimum specimen size is 1 mL.

Special Specimens

For tumor/tissue and various fluids (e.g., CSF, peritoneal fluid, synovial fluid) contact ISI for requirements and special handling instructions.

Shipping Instructions

Specimens should be shipped frozen in dry ice.

References

1. Redfern JS, Feldman M. Role of endogenous prostaglandins in preventing gastrointestinal ulceration: induction of ulcers by antibodies to prostaglandins. Gastroenterology. Feb;96(2 Pt 2 Suppl):596-605, 1989.
2. Bennegard B, Hahlin M, Hamberger L. Luteotropic effects of prostaglandins I_2 and D_2 on isolated human corpora luteum. Fertil Steril. Sep;54(3):459-64, 1990.

CPT Code:
Prostaglandin $F_2\alpha$ 84150

PROSTAGLANDIN $F_2\alpha$ DIHYDROKETO (DHK-$PGF_2\alpha$)

Reference Range

10–50 pg/mL
Reference range is listed on individual patient test reports.

Procedure

DHK-$PGF_2\alpha$ is measured by direct radioimmunoassay/EIA/ELISA.

Patient Preparation

The patient should not take aspirin, indomethacin, or anti-inflammatory medications, if possible, for at least 48 hours prior to collection of specimen.

Specimen Collection

Collect 3 mL serum or EDTA plasma and separate as soon as possible. Freeze serum or plasma immediately after separation. Minimum specimen size is 1 mL.

Special Specimens

For tumor/tissue and various fluids (e.g., CSF, peritoneal fluid, synovial fluid) contact ISI for requirements and special handling instructions.

Shipping Instructions

Specimens should be shipped frozen in dry ice.

References

1. Redfern JS, Feldman M. Role of endogenous prostaglandins in preventing gastrointestinal ulceration: induction of ulcers by antibodies to prostaglandins. Gastroenterology. Feb;96(2 Pt 2 Suppl):596-605, 1989.
2. Strickland DM, Brennecke SP, Mitchell MD. Measurement of 13,14-dihydro-15-keto-prostaglandin F2 alpha and 6-keto-prostaglandin F1 alpha in plasma by radioimmunoassay without prior extraction or chromatography. Prostaglandins Leukot Med. Nov;9(5):491-3, 1982.

CPT Code:
Prostaglandin $F_2\alpha$ 84150

Secretin

Reference Range

12–75 pg/mL
Reference range is listed on individual patient test reports.

Procedure

Secretin is measured by direct radioimmunoassay.

Patient Preparation

The patient should fast for 10 to 12 hours prior to collection of specimen. Antacid medications and medications that affect intestinal motility should be discontinued, if possible, for at least 48 hours prior to collection of specimen.

Specimen Collection

Collect 10 mL EDTA plasma in a special tube containing the GI Preservative and separate as soon as possible. Freeze plasma immediately after separation. Special GI Preservative tubes are available from ISI. Minimum specimen size is 1 mL.

Important Precaution

Secretin specimens must be collected using the GI Preservative tube. No other specimens are acceptable.

Special Specimens

For tumor/tissue and various fluids (e.g., CSF, peritoneal fluid, synovial fluid) contact ISI for requirements and special handling instructions.

Shipping Instructions

Specimens should be shipped frozen in dry ice.

References

1. Christ A, Werth B, Hildebrand P. Human secretin: biologic effects and plasma kinetics in humans. Gastroenterology. Feb;94(2):311-6, 1988.
2. Yanaihara N, Sakagami M, Sato H, et al. Immunological aspects of secretin, substance P and VIP. Apr;72(4 Pt. 2):803-10, 1977.
3. Noda T, Ishikawa O, Eguchi H, et al. [The diagnosis of pancreatic endocrine tumors.] Nippon Rinsho. 62(5):907-10, 2004.
4. Hirst BH. Secretin and the exposition of hormonal control. J Physiol. 15 Oct;560(Pt 2):339, 2004.
5. Chey WY, Chang TM. Secretin, 100 years later. J Gastroenterol. 38(11):1025-35, 2003.
6. Chey WY, Chang TM. Neural control of the release and action of secretin. J Physiol Pharmacol. Dec;54(Suppl 4): 105-12, 2003.
7. Konturek PC, Konturek SJ. The history of gastrointestinal hormones and the Polish contribution to elucidation of their biology and relation to nervous system. J Physiol Pharmacol. 54(Suppl 3):83-98, 2003.

CPT Code:
Unspecified Quantitative Immunoassay 83519

Serotonin (5-HT), Serum

Reference Range

12–44 pg/mL
Reference range is listed on individual patient test reports.

Procedure

Serotonin is measured by direct radioimmunoassay.

Patient Preparation

The patient should fast for 10 to 12 hours prior to collection of specimen. Because of the diurnal variation of serotonin secretion, morning specimens are preferred.

Specimen Collection

Collect 5 mL serum. Separate and freeze serum immediately after separation.
Minimum specimen size is 1 mL.

Important Precaution

For serotonin measurements, avoid hemolysis. Do not use a tourniquet. Handle specimens gently. Hemolysis results in spuriously high results.

Special Specimens

For tumor/tissue and various fluids (e.g., CSF, peritoneal fluid, synovial fluid) contact ISI for requirements and special handling instructions.

Shipping Instructions

Serum specimens should be shipped frozen in dry ice.

References

1. Chauveau J, Fert V, Morel AM, et al. Rapid and specific enzyme immunoassay of serotonin. Clin Chem. 37:1178-84, 1991.
2. Kellum JM Jr, Jaffe BM. Validation and application of a radioimmunoassay for serotonin. Gastroenterology. Apr;70(4):516-22, 1976.
3. Donaldson D. Carcinoid tumours--the carcinoid syndrome and serotonin (5-HT): a brief review. J R Soc Health. Jun;120(2):78-9, 2000.

CPT Code:
Serotonin 84260

SOMATOSTATIN (SOMATOTROPIN RELEASE–INHIBITING FACTOR [SRIF])

Reference Range

Up to 25 pg/mL
Reference range is listed on individual patient test reports.

Procedure

SRIF is measured by direct radioimmunoassay.

Patient Preparation

The patient should fast for 10 to 12 hours prior to collection of specimen. The patient should not take any medications that affect insulin secretion or intestinal motility, if possible, for at least 48 hours prior to collection of specimen.

Specimen Collection

Collect 10 mL EDTA plasma in special tube containing the Z-tube™ Preservative and separate as soon as possible. Freeze plasma immediately after separation. Special Z-tube™ Preservative is available from ISI. Minimum specimen size is 1 mL.

Important Precaution

SRIF specimens must be collected using the GI Preservative tube. No other specimens are acceptable.

Special Specimens

For tumor/tissue and various fluids (e.g., CSF, peritoneal fluid, synovial fluid) contact ISI for requirements and special handling instructions.

Shipping Instructions

Specimens should be shipped frozen in dry ice.

References

1. Vinik AI, Gaginella TS, O'Dorisio TM, et al. The distribution and characterization of somatostatin-like immunoreactivity (SRIF-LI) in isolated cells, submucosa and muscle of the rat stomach and intestine. Endocrinology. Dec;109(6):1921-6, 1981.
2. Hansen BC, Vinik A, Jen KL, et al. Fluctuations in basal levels and effects of altered nutrition on plasma somatostatin. Am J Physiol. Sep;243(3):R289-95, 1982.
3. Lamberts SW. The role of somatostatin in the regulation of anterior pituitary hormone secretion and the use of its analogs in the treatment of human pituitary tumors. Endocr Rev. Nov;9(4):417-36, 1988.
4. Shoelson SE, Polonsky KS, Nakabayashi T. Circulating forms of somatostatinlike immunoreactivity in human plasma. Am J Physiol. Apr;250(4 Pt 1):E428-34, 1986.
5. Low MJ. Clinical endocrinology and metabolism. The somatostatin neuroendocrine system: physiology and clinical relevance in gastrointestinal and pancreatic disorders. Best Pract Res Clin Endocrinol Metab. 18(4):607-22, 2004.

CPT Code:
Somatostatin 84307

SUBSTANCE P

Reference Range

40–270 pg/mL
Reference range is listed on individual patient test reports.

Procedure

Substance P is measured by direct radioimmunoassay.

Patient Preparation

The patient should fast 10 to 12 hours prior to collection of specimen. Antacid medications and medications that affect intestinal motility should be discontinued, if possible, for at least 48 hours prior to collection of specimen.

Specimen Collection

Collect 3 mL serum or EDTA plasma and separate as soon as possible. Substance P is stable at room temperature for 3 days. Specimens can be stored at ambient temperature, refrigerated, or frozen in dry ice. Minimum specimen size is 1 mL.

Special Specimens

For tumor/tissue and various fluids (e.g., CSF, peritoneal fluid, synovial fluid) contact ISI for requirements and special handling instructions.

Shipping Instructions

Specimen can be shipped at ambient temperature, refrigerated, or frozen in dry ice.

References

1. Aronin N, Leeman SE, Clements RS Jr. Diminished flare response in neuropathic diabetic patients: comparison of effects of substance P, histamine and capsaicin. Diabetes. Oct;36(10):1139-43, 1987.
2. Aronin N, Coslovsky R, Chase K. Hypothyroidism increases substance P concentrations in the heterotropic anterior pituitary. Endocrinology. Jun;122(6):2911-4, 1988.
3. Vinik AI, Gonin J, England BG, et al. Plasma substance-P in neuroendocrine tumors and idiopathic flushing: the value of pentagastrin stimulation tests and the effects of somatostatin analog. J Clin Endocrinol Metab. 70(6):1702-9, 1990.

CPT Code:
Unspecified Quantitative Immunoassay 83519

Thyroid-Stimulating Hormone (TSH; Thyrotropin)

Reference Range

0.3–5.0 μU/mL
Reference range is listed on individual patient test reports.

Procedure

TSH is measured by direct radioimmunoassay.

Patient Preparation

The patient should not take any thyroid, steroid, ACTH, estrogen, or corticosteroid medications, if possible, for at least 48 hours prior to collection of specimen.

Specimen Collection

Collect 3 mL serum or EDTA plasma and separate as soon as possible. Freeze plasma immediately after separation. Minimum specimen size is 1 mL.

Special Specimens

For tumor/tissue and various fluids (e.g., CSF, peritoneal fluid, synovial fluid) contact ISI for requirements and special handling instructions.

Shipping Instructions

Specimens should be shipped frozen in dry ice.

References

1. Weintraub BD, Stannard BS, Magner JA, et al. Glycosylation and posttranslational processing of thyroid-stimulating hormone: clinical implications. Recent Prog Horm Res. 41:577-606, 1985.
2. Price A, Griffiths H, Morris BW. A longitudinal study of thyroid function in pregnancy. Clin Chem. Feb;35(2):275-8, 1989.

CPT Code:
Thyroid Stimulating Hormone 84443

THYROTROPIN-RELEASING HORMONE (TRH)

Reference Range

Up to 40 pg/mL
Reference range is listed on individual patient test reports.

Procedure

TRH is measured by direct radioimmunoassay.

Patient Preparation

The patient should not take any thyroid medication, if possible, for at least 48 hours prior to collection of specimen.

Specimen Collection

Collect 5 mL EDTA plasma in a special TRH Preservative tube and separate as soon as possible. Freeze plasma immediately after separation. Special TRH Preservative tubes are available from ISI. Minimum specimen size is 1 mL.

Important Precaution

TRH must be collected with the TRH Preservative tube. No other specimen is acceptable.

Special Specimens

For tumor/tissue and various fluids (e.g., CSF, peritoneal fluid, synovial fluid) contact ISI for requirements and special handling instructions.

Shipping Instructions

Specimens should be shipped frozen in dry ice.

References

1. Kaplan MM, Taft JA, Reichlin S, et al. Sustained rises in serum thyrotropin, thyroxine, and triiodothyronine during long term, continuous thyrotropin-releasing hormone treatment in patients with amyotrophic lateral sclerosis. J Clin Endocrinol Metab. Oct;63(4):808-14, 1986.
2. Shambaugh GE III, Wilber JF, Montoya E, et al. Thyrotropin-releasing hormone (TRH): measurement in human spinal fluid. J Clin Endocrinol Metab. Jul;41(1):131-4, 1975.

CPT Code:
Unspecified Quantitative Immunoassay 83519

THROMBOXANE A_2

Reference Range

180–420 pg/mL
Reference range is listed on individual patient test reports.

Procedure

Thromboxane A_2 is measured by radioimmunoassay of its stable metabolite Thromboxane B_2 following extraction of specimens.

Patient Preparation

The patient should not take aspirin, indomethacin, or anti-inflammatory medications for at least 48 hours prior to collection of specimen. Fasting patients may have elevated levels of thromboxane A_2 metabolite.

Specimen Collection

Collect 3 mL EDTA plasma and separate as soon as possible. Freeze plasma immediately after separation. Minimum specimen size is 1 mL.

Special Specimens

For tumor/tissue and various fluids (e.g., CSF, peritoneal fluid, synovial fluid) contact ISI for requirements and special handling instructions.

Shipping Instructions

Specimens should be shipped frozen in dry ice.

References

1. Clarke RJ, Mayo G, Price P, et al. Suppression of thromboxane A_2 but not of systemic prostacyclin by controlled-release aspirin. N Engl J Med. Oct 17;325(16):1137-41, 1991.
2. Willerson JT, Eidt JF, McNatt J, et al. Role of thromboxane and serotonin as mediators in the development of spontaneous alterations in coronary blood flow and neointimal proliferation in canine models with chronic coronary artery stenoses and endothelial injury. J Am Coll Cardiol. May;17(6 Suppl B):101B-10B, 1991.

CPT Code:
Unspecified Quantitative Immunoassay 83519

THROMBOXANE B_2

Reference Range

180–420 pg/mL
Reference range is listed on individual patient test reports.

Procedure

Thromboxane B_2 is measured by radioimmunoassay following extraction of specimens.

Patient Preparation

The patient should not take aspirin, indomethacin, or anti-inflammatory medications for at least 48 hours prior to collection of specimen. Fasting patients may have elevated levels of thromboxane B_2.

Specimen Collection

Collect 3 mL EDTA plasma and separate as soon as possible. Freeze plasma immediately after separation. Minimum specimen size is 1 mL.

Special Specimens

For tumor/tissue and various fluids (e.g., CSF, peritoneal fluid, synovial fluid) contact ISI for requirements and special handling instructions.

Shipping Instructions

Specimens should be shipped frozen in dry ice.

References

1. Gonzalez-Revalderia J, Sabater J, et al. Usefulness of thromboxane B_2 in diagnosis of renal transplant rejection. Clin Chem. Dec;37(12):2157, 1991.
2. Willerson JT, Eidt JF, McNatt J, et al. Role of thromboxane and serotonin as mediators in the development of spontaneous alterations in coronary blood flow and neointimal proliferation in canine models with chronic coronary artery stenoses and endothelial injury. J Am Coll Cardiol. May;17(6 Suppl B):101B-10B, 1991.

CPT Code:
Unspecified Quantitative Immunoassay 83519

THROMBOXANE B_2, URINE

Reference Range

50–160 ng/24 hours
Reference range is listed on individual patient test reports.

Procedure

Thromboxane B_2 is measured by radioimmunoassay following extraction of specimens.

Patient Preparation

The patient should not take aspirin, indomethacin, or anti-inflammatory medications for at least 48 hours prior to collection of specimen. Fasting patients may have elevated levels of Thromboxane B_2.

Specimen Collection

Submit 5 mL of a 24-hour urine collection. No special preservatives are required. Minimum specimen size is 1 mL. Provide total volume per 24 hours, if possible; random urine samples are acceptable.

Shipping Instructions

Specimens should be shipped frozen in dry ice.

References

1. Gonzalez-Revalderia J, Sabater J, Villafruela JJ, et al. Usefulness of thromboxane B_2 in diagnosis of renal transplant rejection. Clin Chem. Dec;37(12):2157, 1991.
2. Willerson JT, Eidt JF, McNatt J, et al. Role of thromboxane and serotonin as mediators in the development of spontaneous alterations in coronary blood flow and neointimal proliferation in canine models with chronic coronary artery stenoses and endothelial injury. J Am Coll Cardiol. May;17(6 Suppl B):101B-10B, 1991.

CPT Code:
Unspecified Quantitative Immunoassay 83519

VASOACTIVE INTESTINAL POLYPEPTIDE (VIP)

Reference Range

Up to 36 pg/mL
Reference range is listed on individual patient test reports.

Procedure

VIP is measured by direct radioimmunoassay.

Patient Preparation

The patient should fast for 10 to 12 hours prior to collection of specimen. Antacid medications and medications that affect intestinal motility should be discontinued, if possible, for at least 48 hours prior to collection of specimen.

Specimen Collection

Collect 10 mL EDTA plasma in a special tube containing the GI Preservative and separate as soon as possible. Freeze plasma immediately after separation. Special GI Preservative tubes are available from ISI. Minimum specimen size is 1 mL.

Important Precaution

VIP specimens must be collected using the GI Preservative tube. No other specimens are acceptable.

Special Specimens

For tumor/tissue and various fluids (e.g., CSF, peritoneal fluid, synovial fluid) contact ISI for requirements and special handling instructions.

Shipping Instructions

Specimens should be shipped frozen in dry ice.

References

1. O'Dorisio MS, Wood CL, O'Dorisio TM. Vasoactive intestinal peptide and neuropeptide modulation of the immune response. J Immunol. Aug;135(2 Suppl):792S-6S, 1985.
2. Ollerenshaw S, Jarvis D, Woolcock A, et al. Absence of immunoreactive vasoactive intestinal polypeptide in tissue from the lungs of patients with asthma. N Engl J Med. 11 May;320(19):1244-8, 1989.
3. Palsson OS, Morteau O, Bozymski EM, et al. Elevated vasoactive intestinal peptide concentrations in patients with irritable bowel syndrome. Dig Dis Sci. 49(7-8):1236-43, 2004.
4. Gomariz RP, Martinez C, Abad C, et al. Immunology of VIP: a review and therapeutical perspectives. Curr Pharm Des. 7(2):89-111, 2001.
5. Gozes I, Furman S. Clinical endocrinology and metabolism. Potential clinical applications of vasoactive intestinal peptide: a selected update. Best Pract Res Clin Endocrinol Metab. 18(4):623-40, 2001.
6. Kodali S, Ding W, Huang J, et al. Vasoactive intestinal peptide modulates langerhans cell immune function. J Immunol. 173(10):6082-88, 2004.

CPT Code:
Vasoactive Intestinal Polypeptide 84686

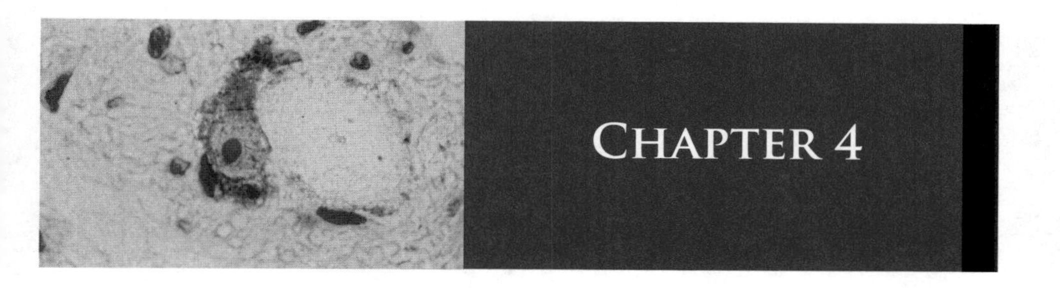

Chapter 4

Profiles, Including CPT Codes

ADENOCARCINOMA OF THE PANCREAS

Ductal adenocarcinoma of the pancreas accounts for 90% of pancreatic cancers. Imaging investigation using CT, with or without fine needle aspiration and assays for tumor and genetic markers, is the primary approach in evaluating patients with symptoms suggestive of pancreatic cancer. Most tumor markers have limited sensitivity and specificity.

BLOOD
- CA 19-9
- CEA

OTHER RELATED TESTS
- Islet amyloid polypeptide (IAPP)
- Glucose
- Glucose tolerance test
- KRAS mutation in pancreatic juice

Patient Preparation

None for blood test.

Specimen Collection

BLOOD
Collect 10 mL serum or EDTA plasma and separate as soon as possible. Freeze serum or plasma immediately after separation. Minimum specimen size is 2 mL.

Shipping Instructions

Specimens should be shipped frozen in dry ice.

References

1. Sawabu N, Watanabe H, Yamaguchi Y, et al. Serum tumor markers and molecular biological diagnosis in pancreatic cancer. Pancreas. Apr;28(3):263-7, 2004.
2. Saisho H, Yamaguchi T. Diagnostic imaging for pancreatic cancer: computed tomography, magnetic resonance imaging, and positron emission tomography. Pancreas. Apr;28(3):273-8, 2004.
3. Chari ST, Klee GG, Miller LJ, et al. Islet amyloid polypeptide is not a satisfactory marker for detecting pancreatic cancer. Gastroenterology. Sep;121(3):640-5, 2001.
4. Rosty C, Goggins M. Early detection of pancreatic carcinoma. Hematol Oncol Clin North Am. Feb;16(1):37-52, 2002.

CPT Codes: Blood
CA 19-9 86301
CEA 82378
CPT Codes: Other Related Tests
Glucose 82947
Glucose Tolerance 82951
IAPP

BRONCHOSPASM PROFILE

This profile is useful for ruling out a neuroendocrine tumor cause of bronchospasm.

BLOOD

- Prostaglandin D_2
- Histamine
- Serotonin
- Substance P
- VIP
- CGA
- Pancreastatin
- Serum protein immunoelectrophoresis, IgE

URINE

- 5-HIAA
- 5-HTP
- VMA
- Tryptase

Patient Preparation

The patient should fast for 10 to 12 hours prior to collection of specimen. Alkali antacid medications should be discontinued, if possible, for at least 24 hours prior to collection. PPIs and H_2 blockers should be discontinued for 72 hours or more prior to collection and patients monitored closely. For 48 hours prior to sample collection, patients should not be treated with the following medications, if possible:

- Insulin or oral medications that influence insulin production or secretion
- Aspirin, indomethacin, or anti-inflammatory medications
- Antacids or medications affecting intestinal motility

Patients should not partake of the following foods for 48 hours prior to collection of urine for measurement of 5-HIAA and 5-HTP:

- Red wine
- Cheese
- Hot dogs
- Chocolates
- Vanilla-containing foods (e.g., ice cream)
- Custard
- Pineapple, kiwi, bananas, or cassava

Specimen Requirements

BLOOD
Collect 10 mL EDTA plasma in special tube containing the Z-tube™ Preservative and separate as soon as possible. Freeze plasma immediately after separation. Special Z-tube™ Preservative is available from ISI. Minimum specimen size is 5 mL.

URINE
See complete urine collection instructions in the introduction to Chapter 3.

Shipping Instructions

Specimens should be shipped frozen in dry ice.

Further Diagnosis

Refer patient for allergy testing.

Reference

1. Chughtai TS, Morin JE, Sheiner NM, et al. Bronchial Carcinoid—20 years experience defines a selective surgical approach. Surgery. Oct;122(4):801-8, 1997.

CPT Codes: Blood
Prostaglandin D_2 84150
Histamine 83088
Serotonin 84260
Substance P 83159
VIP 84686
Chromogranin A 86316
Pancreastatin 83519
Serum Protein Immunoelectrophoresis, IgE 86003
CPT Codes: Urine
5-HIAA Random Urine 83497, 82570
5-HIAA 24-Hour Urine 83497
5-HTP 86701
Vanillyl mandelic acid (VMA) 84585
Tryptase 83520

Carcinoid Follow-Up Profile

BLOOD
Measure every 3 months or immediately following a therapeutic intervention.
- CGA
- Serotonin
- Pancreastatin

If on Sandostatin LAR® for at least three months, consider (measure immediately prior to the LAR® injection):
- Octreotide

For increase in tumor growth or rise in biomarkers, consider other amines, peptides, and markers found to be elevated in the screening evaluation profile, including the following:
- Substance P
- NKA

URINE
Measure every 3 months or immediately following a therapeutic intervention.
- 5-HIAA (or 5-HTP if 5-HIAA is negative and 5-HTP is positive at initial screening)

Patient Preparation

Patient should fast overnight prior to collection of blood specimens. Because of the diurnal variation of serotonin secretion, morning specimens are preferred. For the pancreastatin assay, patients should be advised to discontinue medications that affect insulin levels, if possible, for 48 hours prior to collection. Patients should not partake of the following foods for 48 hours prior to collection of urine for measurement of 5-HIAA and 5-HTP:
- Red wine
- Cheese
- Hot dogs
- Chocolates
- Vanilla-containing foods (e.g., ice cream)
- Custard
- Pineapple, kiwi, bananas, cassava

Specimen Requirements

BLOOD
Collect 10 mL EDTA plasma in special tube containing the Z-tube™ Preservative and separate as soon as possible. Freeze plasma immediately after separation. Special Z-tube™ Preservative is available from ISI. Minimum specimen size is 5 mL. For serotonin analysis, use a yellow-topped tube containing 75 mg ascorbic acid (vitamin C). Separate and freeze plasma immediately.

URINE
See complete urine collection instructions in the introduction to Chapter 3.

Important Precaution

For serotonin measurements, avoid hemolysis. Do not use a tourniquet. Handle specimens gently. Use 20-gauge needle. Hemolysis results in spuriously high results.

Shipping Instructions

Specimens should be shipped frozen in dry ice.

References

1. Oberg K, Kvols L, Caplin M, et al. Consensus report of the use of somatostatin analogs for the management of neuroendocrine tumors of the gastroenteropancreatic system. Ann Oncol. Jun;15(6):966-73, 2004.
2. Please refer to www.nccn.org, The National Comprehensive Cancer Network clinical practice guidelines in oncology.

CPT Codes: Blood
Chromogranin A 86316
Serotonin 84260
Pancreastatin 83519
Octreotide 80299
Neurokinin A 83519
Substance P 83519
CPT Codes: Urine
5-HIAA Random Urine 83497, 82570
5-HIAA 24-Hour Urine 83497
5-HTP 86701

DIABETES TYPE 1 SCREEN

General Screen

General screen tests may be ordered from the local laboratory in each physician's area.

BLOOD

- Glucose
  - Fasting
  - Postprandial
  - Glucose tolerance test

Specific Screening

Specific screening tests are available from ISI.

BLOOD

- Insulin
- C-peptide
- Anti-insulin antibody
- Islet cell antibody
- GAD antibodies (GAD 65, GAD 67)

Patient Preparation

Patient should fast for 10 to 12 hours prior to collection of specimen. Patient should not be on any insulin therapy or taking medications that influence insulin levels, if possible, for at least 48 hours prior to collection of specimen.

Specimen Collection

Collect 10 mL serum or EDTA plasma and separate as soon as possible. Freeze serum or plasma immediately after separation. Minimum specimen size is 2 mL.

Shipping Instructions

Specimens should be shipped frozen in dry ice.

References

1. Skyler JS. New diabetes criteria and clinical implications. Drugs. 58 Suppl 1:1-2, discussion 75-82, 1999.
2. Barker JM, Goehrig SH, Barriga K, et al. DAISY study. Clinical characteristics of children diagnosed with type 1 diabetes through intensive screening and follow-up. Diabetes Care. Jun;27(6):1399-404, 2004.
3. Devendra D, Liu E, Eisenbarth GS. Type 1 diabetes: recent developments. BMJ. 27 Mar;328(7442):750-4, 2004.
4. Eisenbarth GS. Prediction of type 1 diabetes: the natural history of the prediabetic period. Adv Exp Med Biol. 552:268-90, 2004.
5. Pugliese A, Eisenbarth GS. Type 1 diabetes mellitus of man: genetic susceptibility and resistance. Adv Exp Med Biol. 552:170-203, 2004.
6. Krischer JP, Cuthbertson DD, Yu L, et al. Screening strategies for the identification of multiple antibody-positive relative of individuals with type 1 diabetes. J Clin Endocrinol Metab. Jan;88(1):103-8, 2003.
7. Atkinson MA, Eisenbarth GS. Type 1 diabetes: new perspectives on disease pathogenesis and treatment. Lancet. 21 Jul;358(9277):221-9, 2001.
8. Bingley PJ, Bonifacio E, Ziegler AG, et al. Proposed guidelines on screening for risk of type 1 diabetes. Diabetes Care. Feb;24(2):398, 2001.

CPT Codes:
Diabetes Mellitus Type 1 Autoantibody Evaluation 83519, 86337, 86341x2
Hemoglobin A1c 83036
Glucose 82947 • Glucose Tolerance Test 82951 • Glucose Tolerance Test (each additional beyond three specimens) 82952
Insulin 80422, 80432–80435 • Blood 83525 • Free 83527
C-Peptide 80432, 84681
Anti-insulin Antibodies 86337
GAD Antibodies 83519

DIABETES TYPE 2 SCREEN

Predictors of the Development of Type 2 Diabetes

BLOOD

- Lipoprotein profile (either VAP™ or nuclear magnetic resonance [NMR] method)
  - Triglycerides
  - Total cholesterol
  - HDL-C
  - Low-density lipoprotein (LDL)-C
  - LDL-C particle size
- Peptides and cytokines
  - Insulin
  - IL-6
  - C-peptide
  - C-reactive protein (highly sensitive for macrovascular disease)

Patient Preparation

Patient should fast for 10 to 12 hours prior to collection of specimen. Patient should not be on aspirin, pain killers, corticosteroids, indomethacin, or anti-inflammatory medications for at least 48 hours prior to collection of specimen.

CPT Codes:
Insulin 80422, 80432–80435 • Antibody 86337 • Blood 83525 • Free 83527
C-Peptide 80432, 84681
Highly Sensitive C-Reactive Protein (HS CRP) 86140–86141
IL-6 83519
Lipoprotein Profile (VAP™) • Lipoprotein Profile 82465, 84478, 82664, 83700, 83701, 83704, 83718 • VAP™ 83700, 83701, 83704, 84311
Triglycerides 84478
HDL-C 83718
LDL-C 83721

Specimen Collection

Collect 10 mL serum or EDTA plasma and separate as soon as possible. Freeze plasma immediately after separation. Specimens should not be thawed. Minimum specimen size is 6 mL.

Shipping Instructions

Specimens should be shipped frozen in dry ice.

Assessment for Risk Factors for Atherosclerotic Vascular Disease

BLOOD

- Lipoprotein profile (either VAP™ or NMR method)
  - Triglycerides
  - Total cholesterol
  - HDL-C
  - LDL-C
  - LDL-C particle size
- Arachidonic acid/EPA ratio
- Glucose
- HBA1c
- Fibrinogen
- PAI-1
- Thromboglobulin
  - Homocysteine
- C-reactive protein
- IL-6
- Thromboxane B_2

Patient Preparation

Patient should not be on aspirin, pain killers, corticosteroids, indomethacin, or anti-inflammatory medications for at least 48 hours prior to collection of specimens. Fasting patients may have elevated levels of thromboxane B_2.

Specimen Collection

BLOOD
Collect 10 mL serum or EDTA plasma and separate as soon as possible. Freeze plasma immediately after separation. Specimens should not be thawed. Minimum specimen size is 6 mL.

Shipping Instructions

Specimens should be shipped frozen in dry ice.

References

1. Schriger DL, Lorber B. Lowering the cut off point for impaired fasting glucose: where is the evidence? Where is the logic? Diabetes Care. Feb; 27(2):592-601, 2004.
2. Genuth S, Alberti KG, Bennett P, et al. Follow-up report on the diagnosis of diabetes mellitus. Diabetes Care. Nov;26(11):3160-7, 2003.

VAP™ Atherotech, Birmingham, AL 35211

CPT Codes:
Hemoglobin A1c 83036
Insulin 80422, 80432–80435 • Antibody 86337 • Blood 83525 • Free 83527
C-Peptide 80432, 84681
Highly Sensitive C-Reactive Protein (HS CRP) 86140–86141
IL-6 83519
Lipoprotein Profile (VAP™) • Lipoprotein Profile 82465, 84478, 82664, 83700, 83701, 83704, 83718 • VAP™ 83704, 83700, 83701, 84311
Triglycerides 84478
HDL-C 83718
LDL-C 83721
PAI-1 85420-85421
Fibrinogen 85384-85385
Glucose 82947
Homocystine 83090
Homocystine, Urine 82615
Thromboxane B_2 83519
Thromboglobulin 84999
Arachidonic Acid 84999

DIABETES COMPLICATIONS

Gastroparesis or Brittle Diabetes

BLOOD

- Gastrin
- B_{12}
- Gastric parietal cell antibody
- Pancreatic polypeptide (consider meal-stimulated PP measurements or insulin-stimulated PP measurements; see Chapter 5, Meal (Sham Feeding) Stimulation for Vagal Integrity)
- TSH (thyrotoxicosis)
- GH (anorexia nervosa)
- Cortisol (anorexia nervosa, Addison's disease)
- IGF-1 (anorexia nervosa)
- Catecholamines, VMA, and metanephrines (i.e., pheochromocytoma panel)

Patient Preparation

Patient should fast for 10 to 12 hours prior to collection of specimen.

Specimen Collection

Collect 10 mL serum or EDTA plasma and separate as soon as possible. Freeze serum or plasma immediately after separation. Minimum specimen size is 1 mL.

Shipping Instructions

Specimens should be shipped frozen in dry ice.

References

1. Johnson DA, Vinik AI. Gastrointestinal Disturbances. In: Lebovitz HE, ed. Therapy for Diabetes Mellitus and Related Disorders, 4th ed. Alexandria, VA: American Diabetes Association, Inc.; 2004:388-405.
2. Zimmet P, Alberti KG, Shaw J. Global and societal implications of the diabetes epidemic. Nature. 414:782-7, 2004.
3. Ford ES, Giles WH, Dietz WH. Prevalence of the metabolic syndrome among US adults: findings from the third National Health and Nutrition Examination Survey. JAMA. 287:356-9, 2002.
4. Carey VJ, Walters EE, Colditz GA, Solomon CG, Willett WC, Rosner BA, Speizer FE, Manson JE. Body fat distribution and risk of non-insulin-dependent diabetes mellitus in women. The Nurses' Health Study. Am J Epidemiol. 1 Apr;145(7):614-9, 1997.
5. Assmann G, Carmena R, Cullen P, Fruchart JC, Jossa F, Lewis B, Mancini M, Paoletti R. Coronary heart disease: a worldwide view. International Task Force for the Prevention of Coronary Heart Disease. Circulation. 2 Nov;100(18):1930-8, 1999.
6. Gaede P, Vedel P, Larsen N, Jensen GV, Parving HH, Pedersen O. Multifactorial intervention and cardiovascular disease in patients with type 2 diabetes. N Engl J Med. 348:383-93, 2003.
7. Vinik A, Flemmer M. Diabetes and macrovascular disease. J Diabetes Complications. 16:235-45, 2002.
8. National Diabetes Data Group. Diabetes in America, 2nd ed. NIH Publication No. 95-1468. Bethesda, MD: National Diabetes Data Group of the National Institute of Diabetes and Digestive and Kidney Diseases, National Institutes of Health; 1995.
9. National Eye Institute. Facts about diabetic retinopathy. Available at: www.nei.nih.gov/health/diabetic/retinopathy.asp. Accessed 7 June 2005.
10. American Diabetes Association. Standards of medical care for patients with diabetes mellitus. Diabetes Care. 25:213-29, 2002.
11. American Diabetes Association. Diabetic retinopathy. Diabetes Care Suppl. 25:S90-3, 2002.
12. The effect of intensive treatment of diabetes on the development and progression of long-term complications in insulin-dependent diabetes mellitus. The Diabetes Control and Complications Trial Research Group. N Engl J Med. 30 Sep;329(14):977-86, 1993.
13. Stratton IM, Adler AI, Neil HA, Matthews DR, Manley SE, Cull CA, Hadden D, Turner RC, Holman RR. Association of glycaemia with macrovascular and microvascular complications of type 2 diabetes (UKPDS 35): prospective observational study. BMJ. 321:405-12, 2000.
14. Vinik AI, Park TS, Stansberry KB, Pittenger GL. Diabetic neuropathies. Diabetologia. 43:957-73, 2000.
15. Vinik AI, Erbas T. Recognizing and treating diabetic autonomic neuropathy. Cleve Clin J Med. 68:928-44, 2001.

CPT Codes:
Gastrin 82938-82941
B_{12} 82607
Gastric Parietal Cell Antibody 86255
Pancreatic Polypeptide 83519
TSH 84443
GH 83003
Cortisol 82533
IGF-1 84305
Catecholamines 82384
Vanillyl mandelic acid (VMA) 84585
Metanephrines 82570, 83835
Pheochromocytoma Panel 82382, 82570, 83835

Pseudogastrinoma Syndrome (Atrophic Gastritis With Loss of Acid Inhibition of Gastrin)

BLOOD

- Gastrin (elevated)
- Secretin stimulation test of gastrin

If fasting gastrin level is above 100 pg/mL, order a secretin stimulation test. An increase in gastrin level greater than 100 pg/mL above the normal range denotes a gastrinoma.

- Chromogranin A (not due to a neuroendocrine tumor)
  - May be suspected with mean corpuscular volume greater than 100 μm^3
- B_{12}
- Pepsinogen I and II

Important Precaution

Patients submitted to dynamic challenge should be under the direct and constant supervision of their physician at all times. The doses listed are intended as a guideline only. The actual dose and collection schedule must be approved by the patient's physician.

Specimen Collection

Collect 10 mL serum or EDTA plasma and separate as soon as possible. Freeze serum or plasma immediately after separation. Minimum specimen size is 2 mL.

GASTRIC PH

Patient Preparation

Patient should fast 10 to 12 hours prior to collection of specimen. Alkali antacid medications should be discontinued, if possible, for at least 24 hours prior to collection. PPIs and H_2 blockers should be discontinued for 72 hours or more prior to collection and patients monitored closely.

Shipping Instructions

Specimens should be shipped frozen in dry ice.

CPT Codes:
Gastrin 82938–82941
Chromogranin A 86316
B_{12} 82607
Secretin Stimulation Test 82938
Pepsinogen I 83519
Pepsinogen II 83519

References

1. Owyang C, Vinik AI. Diabetic pseudo Zollinger-Ellison syndrome. Gastroenterol. 82(5):1144, 1982.
2. DuFour DR, Gaskin JH, Jubiz WA. Dynamic procedures in endocrinology. In: Becker KL, ed. Principles and Practice of Endocrinology and Metabolism. Philadelphia: JB Lippincott Company; 1990:1762-75.
3. Alsever RN, Gotlin RW. Handbook of Endocrine Tests in Adults and Children. Chicago: Year Book Medical Publishers, Inc.; 1978.
4. Feldman M, Schiller LR, Walsh JH, et al. Positive intravenous secretin test in patients with achlorhydria-related hypergastrinemia. Gastroenterol. 93:59-62, 1987.

DIARRHEA SYNDROME TESTS

BLOOD

- VIP
- Gastrin
- Gastrin-releasing peptide (bombesin)
- Calcitonin (MCT)
- PGD_2
- Histamine
- CGA
- Pancreastatin
- Pancreatic polypeptide
- PTH and PTHRP if hypercalcemic
- CGRP and substance P if flushing

URINE

- 5-HIAA
- 5-HTP
- VMA and catecholamines if hypertensive

STOOL

Measurement of stool electrolytes and osmolarity should be done early in the diagnostic evaluation. The presence of an osmolar gap suggests factitious diarrhea. A 72-hour supervised fast with intravenous fluid administration may also help determine if the diarrhea is secretory or infectious.

Patient Preparation

Patient should fast for 10 to 12 hours prior to collection of blood specimen. Antacid medications, antihistamine medications, aspirin, indomethacin, anti-inflammatory medications, and medications affecting motility or pancreatic function should be discontinued, if possible, for at least 48 hours prior to collection. Patients should not partake of the following foods for 48 hours prior to collection of urine for measurement of 5-HIAA and 5-HT:

- Red wine
- Cheese
- Hot dogs
- Chocolates
- Vanilla-containing foods (e.g., ice cream)
- Custard
- Pineapple, kiwi, bananas, cassava

Specimen Requirements

BLOOD

Collect 10 mL EDTA plasma in a special tube containing the GI Preservative and separate as soon as possible. Freeze plasma immediately after separation. Special GI Preservative tubes are available from ISI. Minimum specimen size is 1 mL. For other assays that do not require the GI Preservative, 10 mL serum or EDTA plasma may be submitted.

URINE

See complete urine collection instructions in the introduction to (Chapter 3).

Shipping Instructions

Specimens should be shipped frozen in dry ice.

References

1. Vinik AI, Tsai ST, Moattari AR, et al. Somatostatin analogue (SMS 201-995) in the management of gastroenteropancreatic tumors and diarrhea syndromes. Am J Med. 81(6B):23-40, 1986.
2. Verner JV, Morrison AB. Islet cell tumor and a syndrome of refractory watery diarrhea and hypokalemia. Am J Med. 25(3):374-80, 1958.
3. Murray JS, Paton RR, Pope CE. Pancreatic tumor associated with flushing and diarrhea. Report of a case. N Engl J Med. 264:436-9, 1961.
4. Arnold R, Lankisch PG. Somatostatin and the gastrointestinal tract. Clin Gastroenterol. 9(3):733-53, 1980.
5. Stockmann F, Richter G, Lembeke B, Conlon JM, Creutzfeldt W. Long-term treatment of patients with endocrine gastrointestinal tumors with the somatostatin analogue SMS 201-995. Scand J Gastroenterol. 21:230, 1986.
6. Hengl G, Prager J, Pointner H. The influence of somatostatin on the absorption of triglycerides in partially gastrectomized subjects. Acta Hepatogastroenterol (Stuttg). Oct;26(5):392-5, 1979.
7. Vinik A, Moattari AR. Use of somatostatin analog in management of carcinoid syndrome. Dig Dis Sci; 34(3 Suppl):14S-27S, 1989.

CPT Codes: Blood
Vasoactive Intestinal Polypeptide (VIP) 84686
Gastrin 82938-82941
Bombesin 83519
Calcitonin 82308
Prostaglandin D_2 84150
Histamine 83088
Chromogranin A 86316
Pancreastatin 83519
Pancreatic Polypeptide 83519
PTH 83519
PTHRP 83519
CGRP: Unlisted Chemistry Procedure 84999 or Unspecified Immunoassay 83520
Substance P 83519
CPT Codes: Urine
5-HIAA 83497
5-HTP 86701
Vanillyl mandelic acid (VMA) 84585
Catecholamines 82384

Dumping Syndrome

BASAL/FASTING TESTS

Following an overnight fast, patients should have blood drawn for the following tests:

- Pancreatic polypeptide
- Glucagon
- GLP-1
- Insulin
- Motilin
- GIP

FECAL MEASUREMENTS

- Fecal fat measurement
- Fecal chymotrypsin measurement
- Fecal EL1 measurement

Patient Preparation

Patients should fast for 10 to 12 hours prior to collection of specimens. Patients should discontinue medications that affect insulin production or secretion, antacid medications, or medications affecting intestinal motility, if possible, for 48 hours prior to collection.

Specimen Collection

BLOOD

For the glucagon and GIP analyses, collect 3 mL EDTA plasma in a special tube containing the GI Preservative and separate as soon as possible. Freeze plasma immediately after separation. Special GI Preservative tubes are available from ISI. Minimum specimen size is 1 mL.

STOOL

Collect 100 mg of formed stool and store at –20°C. Stool specimens are stable for 7 days at refrigerated temperatures. Minimum specimen size is 20 mg of formed stool. Note on request slip if sample has watery diarrhea consistency, as concentration levels of EL1 may be decreased due to dilution factor.

Shipping Instructions

Specimen should be shipped frozen in dry ice.

References

1. Harris AG, O'Dorisio TM, Woltering EA, et al. Consensus statement: octreotide dose titration in secretory diarrhea. Diarrhea Management Consensus Development Panel. Dig Dis Sci. Jul;40(7):1464-73, 1995.
2. Mozell EJ, Woltering EA, O'Dorisio TM. Non-endocrine applications of somatostatin and octreotide acetate: facts and flights of fancy. Dis Mon. Dec;37(12):749-848, 1991.
3. Richards WO, Geer R, O'Dorisio TM, et al. Octreotide acetate induces fasting small bowel motility in patients with dumping syndrome. J Surg Res. Dec;49(6):483-7, 1990.
4. Geer RJ, Richards WO, O'Dorisio TM, et al. Efficacy of octreotide acetate in treatment of severe postgastrectomy dumping syndrome. Ann Surg. Dec;212(6):678-87, 1990.
5. Woltering EA, O'Dorisio TM, Williams ST, et al. Treatment of nonendocrine gastrointestinal disorders with octreotide acetate. Metabolism. Sep;39(9 Suppl 2):176-9, 1990.

CPT Codes:
GLP-1 83519
Insulin 83525 • Proinsulin 84206 • Proinsulin Serum 84206
Motilin 83519
Amylase 82150
Lipase 83690
Trypsin 84488
Fecal Fat • Quantitative 82710 • Qualitative 82705
Fecal Chymotrypsin 84311
Fecal Elastase I 82656
GIP 83519

FLUSHING SYNDROME TESTS

Tests to Identify Causes of Flushing in Different Clinical Syndromes

Clinical Condition	Tests
Carcinoid	Urine 5-HIAA, 5-HTP, substance P, CGRP, CGA
MCT	Calcitonin, calcium infusion, RET protooncogene
Pheochromocytoma	VMA, epinephrine, norepinephrine, dopamine, glucagon stimulation test, T2-weighted MRI, OctreoScan®, MIBG
Diabetic autonomic neuropathy	Heart rate variability, 2-hour postprandial glucose
Menopause	FSH
Epilepsy	Electroencephalogram
Panic syndrome	Pentagastrin-stimulated ACTH
Mastocytosis	Histamine (plasma), VIP, tryptase (urine)
Hypomastia, mitral prolapse	Echocardiography

BLOOD
- CGA
- Pancreastatin
- Substance P
- VIP
- Gastrin
- Neurotensin
- Serotonin
- CGRP
- Calcitonin
- FSH
- Histamine

URINE

For all 24-hour urine collections, measure creatinine.
- 5-HIAA
- 5-HTP
- VMA if hypertensive
- Tryptase

CONSIDER
- Plasma catecholamines if hypertensive
- Dopamine
- Epinephrine
- Norepinephrine
- PTH and PTHRP if hypercalcemic
- MEN screen (gastrin, prolactin, pancreatic polypeptide, and ionized Ca^{++})
- MEN-I gene and RET protooncogene
- Calcitonin, gastrin, and ACTH for degree of tumor aggression
- CA 19-1
- BNP, otherwise known as atrial natriuretic factor, if echocardiogram abnormal

ADDITIONAL TESTING IN PATIENTS WITH UNUSUAL CLINICAL SYNDROMES

- GHRH
- Bombesin
- Ghrelin
- IGF-1, IGF-2
- Corticotropin-releasing factor (CRF)

TISSUE STAINS

- K167
- CGA
- Synaptophysin
- NSE
- Somatostatin receptor type 2

CONSIDER

- Factor VIII, CD 31, AE1/AE3
- Somatostatin receptor subtypes other than type 2

Patient Preparation

Patient should fast overnight prior to collection of blood specimens. Antacid medications and medications affecting motility should be discontinued, if possible for at least 48 hours prior to collection of specimens. Patients should not partake of the following foods for 48 hours prior to collection of urine for measurement of 5-HIAA and 5-HTP measurements:

- Red wine
- Cheese
- Hot dogs
- Chocolates
- Vanilla-containing foods (e.g., ice cream)
- Custard
- Pineapple, kiwi, bananas, cassava

Specimen Requirements

BLOOD
Collect 20 mL of blood in a green-topped EDTA tube. For serotonin analysis, use a yellow-topped tube containing 75 mg ascorbic acid (vitamin C). Separate and freeze plasma immediately. For bombesin and VIP analyses, collect 5 mL EDTA plasma in a special tube containing the GI Preservative and separate as soon as possible. Freeze plasma immediately after separation. Special GI Preservative tubes are available from ISI. Minimum specimen size is 1 mL.

TISSUE
Consult specialist for tissue staining requirements.

URINE
See complete urine collection instructions in the introduction to Chapter 3.

Shipping Instructions

Specimens should be shipped frozen in dry ice.

References

1. Vinik AI, Tsai ST, Moattari AR, et al. Somatostatin analogue (SMS 201-995) in the management of gastroenteropancreatic tumors and diarrhea syndromes. Am J Med. 81(6B):23-40, 1988.
2. Verner JV, Morrison AB. Islet cell tumor and a syndrome of refractory watery diarrhea and hypokalemia. Am J Med. 25(3):374-80, 1958.
3. Murray JS, Paton RR, Pope CE. Pancreatic tumor associated with flushing and diarrhea. Report of a case. N Engl J Med. 264:436-9, 1961.
4. Arnold R, Lankisch PG. Somatostatin and the gastrointestinal tract. Clin Gastroenterol. 9(3):733-53, 1980.
5. Stockmann F, Richter G, Lembeke B, et al. Long-term treatment of patients with endocrine gastrointestinal tumors with the somatostatin analogue SMS 201-995. Scand J Gastroenterol. 2:230, 1986.
6. Hengl G, Prager J, Pointner H. The influence of somatostatin on the absorption of triglycerides in partially gastrectomized subjects. Acta Hepatogastroenterol (Stuttg). 26(5):392-5, 1979.
7. Vinik A, Moattari AR. Use of somatostatin analog in management of carcinoid syndrome. Dig Dis Sci. 34(3 Suppl): 14S-27S, 1989.

CPT Codes:
Urine • 5-HIAA Random Urine 83497, 82570 • 5-HIAA 24-Hour Urine 83497 • 5-HTP 86701 • VMA 84585 • Tryptase 83520
Calcitonin 82308
Epinephrine 82383
Norepinephrine 82725
FSH 83001
ACTH 82024
Histamine 83088
Substance P 83519
Gastrin 82938-82941
VIP 84686
Neurotensin 83519
Chromogranin A 86316
Calcium 82310
Catecholamines 82384
PTH 83519
PTH RP 83519
BNP 83880
Growth Hormone–Releasing Hormone 83519
Bombesin 83519
IGF-1 84305
IGF-2 83520
Ghrelin 84999 Unlisted Chemistry Procedure
CRF 84999 Unlisted Chemistry Procedure
Enolase 86316
MEN Type I Screen • Gastrin 82938–82941 • Prolactin 84146 • Pancreatic Polypeptide 83519 • Iolonized Calcium 82330
Glucagon 82943 • Tolerance Panel 80422–80424 • Tolerance Test 82946
Insulin 83525 • Proinsulin 84206 • Proinsulin Serum 84206

Gastrinoma (Zollinger-Ellison) Screen

BASAL/FASTING TESTS

- Fasting gastrin concentration
- Gastric pH

CONSIDER

- Pancreatic polypeptide for pancreatic location and suspected MEN-I
- MEN-I screen
- ACTH if rapid tumor growth, history of hypertension, diabetes, bruising, etc.
- OctreoScan and CT or MRI

Patient Preparation

Patient should fast for 10 to 12 hours prior to collection of specimen. Alkali antacid medications should be discontinued, if possible, for at least 24 hours prior to collection. PPIs and H_2 blockers should be discontinued for 72 hours prior to collection and patients monitored closely.

Specimen Collection

Collect 10 mL serum or EDTA plasma and separate as soon as possible. Freeze serum or plasma immediately after separation. Minimum specimen size is 1 mL.

Shipping Instructions

Specimens should be shipped frozen in dry ice.

References

1. Trudeau WI, McGuigan JE. Effects of calcium on serum gastrin levels in the Zollinger-Ellison syndrome. N Engl J Med. 16 Oct;281(16):862-6, 1969.
2. Mozell EJ, Woltering EA, O'Dorisio TM, et al. Effect of somatostatin analog on peptide release and tumor growth in the Zollinger-Ellison syndrome. Surg Gynecol Obstet. Jun;170(6):476-84, 1990.
3. Mozell EJ, Cramer AJ, O'Dorisio TM, et al. Long-term efficacy of octreotide in the treatment of Zollinger-Ellison syndrome. Arch Surg. Sep;127(9):1019-24, discussion 1024-6, 1992.
4. Mignon, M. Diagnostic and therapeutic strategies in Zollinger-Ellison syndrome associated with multiple endocrine neoplasia type I (MEN-I): experience of the Zollinger-Ellison Syndrome Research Group: Bichat 1958-1999. Bull Acad Nat Med. 187(7):1249-58, 2003.
5. Mozell EJ, Woltering EA, O'Dorisio TM, et al. Effect of somatostatin analog on peptide release and tumor growth in the Zollinger-Ellison syndrome. Surg Gynecol Obstet. Jun;170(6):476-84, 1990.
6. Owyang C, Vinik AI. Diabetic pseudo Zollinger-Ellison syndrome. Gastroenterol. 82(5):1144, 1982.

CPT Codes:
Gastrin 82941
ACTH 82024
Pancreatic Polypeptide 83519
MEN Type I Screen • Gastrin 82938–82941 • Prolactin 84146 • Pancreatic Polypeptide 83519 • Ionized Calcium 82330

GENERIC FOLLOW-UP PROFILES PANCREAS AND MEN TESTS

BLOOD

- Ca^{++} corrected for albumin concentrations
- Every 3 months, measure specific peptides found to be elevated on screening profile
- Check other components of MEN syndrome screen for MEN measurements (see previous page)

CONSIDER

- Octreotide suppression test, a predictive test for responsiveness to somatostatin analog therapy
- Octreotide levels for patients on drug, if patient symptoms, tumor, and biochemical markers are not responding
- RET protooncogene and MEN-I gene (MENIN) if not tested previously

Patient Preparation

Patient should fast for 10 to 12 hours prior to collection of specimen. Alkali antacid medications should be discontinued, if possible, for at least 24 hours prior to collection. PPIs and H_2 blockers should be discontinued for 72 hours prior to collection and patients monitored closely.

Specimen Requirements:

For plasma peptides, collect 10 mL whole blood in an EDTA plasma tube. Separate and freeze plasma immediately. For the isolation of DNA for genetic testing, send 10 mL of whole blood in green-topped tube. Do not separate, do not freeze.

Shipping Instructions

Specimens should be shipped frozen in dry ice.

References

1. Mozell EJ, Woltering EA, O'Dorisio TM, et al. Effect of somatostatin analog on peptide release and tumor growth in the Zollinger-Ellison syndrome. Surg Gynecol Obstet. Jun;170(6):476-84, 1990.
2. Mozell EJ, Woltering EA, O'Dorisio TM, et al. Adult onset nesidioblastosis: response of glucose, insulin, and secondary peptides to therapy with Sandostatin. Am J Gastroenterol. Feb;85(2):181-8, 1990.
3. Please refer to www.endotext.org.

CPT Codes:
Octreotide 80299
MEN Type I Screen • Gastrin 82938-82941 • Prolactin 84146 • Pancreatic Polypeptide 83519 • Ionized Calcium 82330

GENETIC STUDIES

Neuroendocrine Tumors

BLOOD

- MEN-I (MENIN gene)
- RET protooncogene (MEN-II)

Type 1 Diabetes

BLOOD

- HLA
- DR3
- DR4
- A_2

Risk Factors for Diabetic Complications

- Superoxide dismutase gene polymorphism
- Toll receptor polymorphism
- ApoE gene polymorphism
- Angiotensin receptor gene polymorphism
- Glut 4 abnormalities
- Hepatic nuclear transcription factor 1 and 4 (MODY)
- Aldose reductase gene polymorphism (Z2 allele)
- Cytochrome P450 polymorphism
- TNFα gene polymorphism
- 5′ Lipoxygenase gene polymorphism
- Mitochondrial DNA mutations
- Glucokinase gene abnormalities
- Mitochondrial DNA

Patient Preparation

Consult specialist for patient preparation.

Specimen Requirements

Consult specialist for specimen requirements.

Shipping Instructions

Consult specialist for shipping instructions.

Reference

1. Please refer to www.endotext.org.

GI–Neuroendocrine Tests

BLOOD

- Neurotensin
- Ghrelin
- PTH
- PTHRP
- Prolactin
- Glucagon
- Insulin (if history of hypoglycemia) IGF I and IGF II
- C-Peptide (if history of hypoglycemia)
- Somatostatin
- Calcitonin
- VIP
- Gastrin
- Catecholamines (dopamine, epinephrine and norepinephrine if hypertensive)

Patient Preparation

Patient should be fasting 10 to 12 hours prior to collection of specimen. Antacid medication, Corticosteroid, ACTH, Thyroid, Estrogen or Gonadotropin medications and medications affecting motility, gastrointestinal or pancreatic function should be discontinued, if possible, for at least 48 hours prior to collection.

URINE

- VMA if hypertensive
- Catecholamines [dopamine, epinephrine, (metaepinephrine) norepinephrine (normetanephrine) if hypertensive]

Specimen Requirements

BLOOD
Collect 10 mL EDTA plasma in a special tube containing the GI Preservative and separate as soon as possible. Freeze plasma immediately after separation. Minimum specimen size is 2 mL. Special GI Preservative tubes are available from ISI for these assays: glucagon, somatostatin, and VIP. Submit 10 mL serum or EDTA plasma for other assays not requiring the GI Preservative.

URINE (FOR CATECHOLAMINES ONLY)
Measure 10 mL of 24-hour urine collection. Minimum specimen size is 2 mL. Random urine samples are acceptable if 24-hour total volume is not available.

Important Precaution

Specimens for assays specified must be collected using the GI Preservative tube. No other specimens are acceptable for these assays.

Shipping Instructions

Specimens should be shipped frozen in dry ice.

References

1. Please refer to www.endotext.org.
2. Please refer to Aaron I. Vinik in www.endotext.org/guthormones/index.htm.

CPT Codes:
Neurotensin 83519
Ghrelin 83519
PTH 83519
PTH-Related Peptide 83519
Prolactin 84146
Glucagon 82943 • Tolerance Panel 80422–80424 • Tolerance Test 82946
Insulin
IGF-1 84305
IGF-2 83520
C-Peptide
Somatostatin 84307
Calcitonin 82308
VIP 84686
Gastrin 82938–82941
Catecholamines 82384
Dopamine 82384
Epinephrine 82383
Norepinephrine 82725
Insulin 80422, 80432–80435 • Antibody 86337 • Blood 83525 • Free 83527

Hypoglycemia/Insulinoma Screening Test

Patient Preparation

Patients should be advised to discontinue medications that affect insulin levels, if possible, for 48 hours prior to collection. After an overnight fast, basal blood samples are collected to measure the following:

- Insulin
- Proinsulin
- C-peptide
- IGF-1 and IGF-2

Specimen Requirements

Collect 6 mL of serum or EDTA plasma and separate as soon as possible. Freeze serum or plasma immediately after separation. Minimum specimen size is 4 mL.

Shipping Instructions

Specimen should be shipped frozen in dry ice.

Reference

1. Fajans SS, Vinik AI. Diagnosis and treatment of "insulinoma." In: Santen RJ, Manni A, eds. Diagnosis and Management of Endocrine-Related Tumors. Boston, MA: Martinus Nijhoff Publishers; 1984:235.

CPT Codes:
Insulin 83525
Proinsulin 84206
Proinsulin Serum 84206
C-Peptide 80432, 84681
IGF-1 84305
IGF-2 83520

Interleukins Individually and as a Profile (IL-1 through IL-18)

Reference Range

See individual assays in Chapter 3.

Procedure

Interleukins are measured by enzyme immunoassay.

Patient Preparation

Patient should not be on any corticosteroids, anti-inflammatory medications, or pain killers, if possible, for at least 48 hours prior to collection.

Specimen Collection

Collect 3 mL serum or EDTA plasma and separate as soon as possible. Freeze specimen immediately after separation. Minimum specimen size is 1 mL.

Important Precaution

The interleukins are unstable in freeze-thaw cycles. Do not thaw prior to shipping; specimens must remain frozen from immediately after collection until assayed.

Special Specimens

For tumor/tissue and various fluids (e.g., CSF, peritoneal fluid, synovial fluid) contact ISI for requirements and special handling instructions.

Shipping Instructions

Specimens should be shipped frozen in dry ice.

References

1. Whicher JT, Evans SW. Cytokines in disease. Clin Chem. 36:1269-81, 1990.
2. Bevilacqua MP, Pober JS, Majeau GR, et al. Recombinant tumor necrosis factor induces procoagulant activity in cultured human vascular endothelium: characterization and comparison with the actions of interleukin 1. Proc Natl Acad Sci USA. Jun;83(12):4533-7, 1986.
3. Huang CM, Elin RJ, Ruddel M, et al. Changes in laboratory results for cancer patients treated with interleukin-2. Clin Chem. Mar;36(3):431-4, 1990.
4. Ihle JN. The molecular and cellular biology of interleukin-3. Year Immunol. 5:59-102, 1989.
5. Galizzi JP, Castle B, Djossou O, et al. Purification of a 130-kDa T cell glycoprotein that binds human interleukin 4 with high affinity. J Biol Chem. Jan 5;265(1):439-44, 1990.
6. Bischoff SC, Brunner T, De Weck AL, et al. Interleukin 5 modifies histamine release and leukotriene generation by human basophils in response to diverse agonists. J Exp Med. 1 Dec;172(6):1577-82, 1990.
7. Spangelo BL, Jarvis WD, Judd AM, et al. Induction of interleukin-6 release by interleukin-1 in rat anterior pituitary cells in vitro: evidence for an eicosanoid-dependent mechanism. Endocrinology. Dec;129(6):2886-94, 1991.
8. Hunt P, Robertson D, Weiss D, et al. A single bone marrow-derived stromal cell type supports the in vitro growth of early lymphoid and myeloid cells. Cell. 27 Mar;48(6):997-1007, 1987.
9. Matsushima K, Oppenheim JJ. Interleukin 8 and MCAF: novel inflammatory cytokines inducible by IL 1 and TNF. Cytokine. Nov;1(1):2-13, 1989.

CPT Codes:
IL-1α, IL-1β or Any Interleukin Through IL-18 83519

LIPOPROTEIN PROFILE (TOTAL CHOLESTEROL, HDL-C, LDL-C, PARTICLE SIZE, AND TRIGLYCERIDES)

Lipoprotein profile (either VAP™ or NMR method)

- Triglycerides
- Total cholesterol
- HDL-C
- LDL-C
- LDL-C particle size

Patient Preparation

Consult local laboratory for patient preparation.

Specimen Requirements

Consult local laboratory for specimen requirements.

Shipping Instructions

Consult local laboratory for shipping instructions.

Reference

1. Please refer to www.endotext.org.

CPT Codes:
HDL-C 83718
LDL-C 83721
Particle Size 82465, 83704
Total Cholesterol 82465
Triglycerides 84478

MEN Syndrome Screen

BLOOD

- Pituitary (MEN-I)
  - Prolactin
  - Growth hormone if features of acromegaly
- Parathyroid (MEN-I and -II)
  - PTH
  - PTHRP
  - Ionized Ca^{++} or Ca^{++} corrected for serum albumin
  - 24-Hour urine collection for Ca^{++} and PO_4
- Pancreas (MEN-I)
  - Pancreatic polypeptide
  - Gastrin
  - Insulin/C-peptide if patient hypoglycemic
  - CGA
- Thyroid C cells (MEN-II)
  - Calcitonin
  - CEA
- Adrenal (MEN-II)
  - Catecholamines (plasma and urine determinations)

URINE

- VMA
- Catecholamines if hypertensive or VMA is positive
- 5-HIAA
- 5-HTP

TISSUE IMMUNOHISTOCHEMISTRY (FORMALIN-FIXED 2-mm^3 SPECIMENS)

- CGA
- NSE
- Synaptophysin
- Ki-67, AE1, and AE3
- Glucagon
- Gastrin
- Insulin
- Somatostatin
- PP
- Consider factor VIII, CD31, and somatostatin receptors

GENETIC SCREENING

- RET protooncogene
- MEN-I gene

Patient Preparation

Patient should fast overnight prior to collection of blood specimens. Antacid medications and medications affecting intestinal motility should be discontinued, if possible, for at least 48 hours prior to collection of specimens. Patients should not partake of the following foods for 48 hours prior to collection of urine for measurement of 5-HIAA and 5-HTP measurements:

- Red wine
- Cheese
- Hot dogs
- Chocolates
- Vanilla-containing foods (e.g., ice cream)
- Custard
- Pineapple, kiwi, bananas, cassava

Specimen Requirements

BLOOD
Collect 20 mL of blood in a green-topped EDTA tube. For serotonin analysis, use a yellow-topped tube containing 75 mg ascorbic acid (vitamin C) for the blood collection. Separate and freeze plasma immediately. For bombesin and VIP analyses, collect 5 mL EDTA plasma in a special tube containing the GI Preservative and separate as soon as possible. Freeze plasma immediately after separation. Special GI Preservative tubes are available from ISI. Minimum specimen size is 1 mL.

TISSUE
Consult specialist for tissue staining requirements.

URINE
See complete urine collection instructions in the introduction to Chapter 3.

Shipping Instructions

Specimens should be shipped frozen in dry ice.

References

1. Please refer to www.endotext.org.
2. Please refer to Roger R. Perry in www.endotext.org/guthormones/index.htm.

CPT Codes: Blood
Pituitary (MEN-I) • Prolactin 84146 • Growth Hormone 83003
Parathyroid (MEN-I and -II) • Parathyroid Hormone (PTH) 83519 • PTHRP 83519 • Ionized Ca^{++} or Ca^{++} Corrected for Serum Albumin 82330
Pancreas (MEN-I) • Pancreatic Polypeptide 83519 • Gastrin 82938–82941 • Insulin 83525 • C-peptide 84681 • Chromogranin A 86316
Thyroid C Cells (MEN-II) • Calcitonin 82308 • Carcinoembryonic Antigen (CEA) 82378
Adrenal (MEN-II) • Catecholamines 82384
CPT Codes: Urine
Vanillyl mandelic acid (VMA) 84585
Catecholamines 82384
5-HIAA 83497, 82570
5-HTP 86701
CPT Codes: Tissue Immunohistochemistry (Formalin-Fixed 2-mm³ Specimens)
Chromogranin A 86316
Neuron-Specific Enolase 86316
Synaptophysin NO CODE AVAILABLE FOR IHC SYNAPTOPHYSIN
Ki-67 NO CODE AVAILABLE FOR IHC Ki-67; Ki-67, Breast Cancer 88360
AE 1 and AE 3 84999 Unlisted Chemistry Procedure
Glucagon NO CODE AVAILABLE FOR IHC GLUCAGON
Glucagon 82943 • Tolerance Panel 80422–80424 • Tolerance Test 82946
Gastrin NO CODE AVAILABLE FOR IHC GASTRIN
Gastrin 82938–82941
Insulin NO CODE AVAILABLE FOR IHC INSULIN BLOCK
Insulin 83525
Somatostatin 84307
Pancreatic Polypeptide 83519

Metabolic Syndrome Profile

- Insulin (1 test)
- Fasting glucose (1 test)
- HOMA index

HOMA IR = Fasting Insulin (μU/mL) x Fasting Glucose (mmol/L)/22.5
HOMA B = Fasting Insulin (μU/mL)/[Fasting Glucose (mmol/L) – 3.5]

- Insulin secretory index

Insulin Secretory Index = [Insulin 30 min (pmol/L) - Insulin 0 min (pmol/L)]/
[Glucose 30 min (mmol/L) – Glucose 0 min (mmol/L)]

- HBA1c (1 test)
- C-peptide (2 tests)
- Free fatty acids (FFAs; 2 tests)
- Highly sensitive C-reactive protein (HS CRP; 1 test)
- PAI-1 (1 test)
- Fibrinogen (1 test)
- Adiponectin (1 test)
- IL-6 (1 test)
- Free and total testosterone (free index; 2 tests)
- Sex steroid–binding globulin (2 tests)
- Uric acid (2 tests)
- Lipoprotein profile (VAP™; 1 test)
- Apolipoproteins (2 test)
- Microalbumin (spot/g creatinine; 1 test)
- Angiotensin I and II
- Endothelin I

Patient Preparation

Patient should fast for 10 to 12 hours prior to collection of specimen. Patient should be on a normal-sodium diet (110 mEq sodium) and recumbent for at least 30 minutes prior to draw. Patient should not be on ACTH, corticosteroid, diuretics, mineralocorticoids, glucocorticoids, estrogens, oral contraceptives, or hypertension medications, if possible, for 48 hours prior to collection.

Specimen Collection

Collect 20 mL EDTA plasma and separate as soon as possible. Freeze plasma immediately after separation. Minimum specimen size is 10 mL.

Shipping Instructions

Specimens should be shipped frozen in dry ice.

References

1. Goodman E, Daniels SR, Morrison JA, et al. Contrasting prevalence of and demographic disparities in the World Health Organization and National Cholesterol Education Program Adult Treatment Panel III definitions of metabolic syndrome among adolescents. J Pediatr. Oct;145(4):445-51, 2004.
2. Grundy SM, Brewer HB Jr, Cleeman JI, et al. Definition of metabolic syndrome: report of the National Heart, Lung, and Blood Institute/American Heart Association conference on scientific issues related to definition. Arterioscler Thromb Vasc Biol. Feb;24(2):13-8, 2004.
3. Mathews DR, Hosker JP, Rudenski AS, et al. Homeostasis model assessment: insulin resistance and beta-cell function from fasting plasma glucose and insulin concentrations in man. Diabetologia. 28:412-9, 1985.

CPT Codes:
Insulin 80422, 80432–80435 • Antibody 86337 • Blood 83525 • Free 83527
Fasting Glucose 82947
HBA1c 83036
C-Peptide 80432, 84681
Free Fatty Acids (FFAs) 82725
Highly Sensitive C-Reactive Protein (HS CRP) 86140–86141
PAI-1 85420–85421
Fibrinogen 85384–85385
Adiponectin 83520, Unspecified Immunoassay
IL-6 83519
Free and Total Testosterone 84402, 84403
Sex Hormone–Binding Globulin 84270
Uric Acid • Uric Acid 84550 • Uric Acid Random/24-Hour 84560
Lipoprotein Profile (VAP™) • Lipoprotein Profile 82465, 84478, 82664, 83716, 83718 • VAP™ 83716, 84311
Apolipoproteins 84478
Microalbumin (spot/g Creatinine) 82043, 82570
Angiotensin I and II • Angiotensin I 82164 • Angiotensin II 82163
Endothelin I 83519

OXIDATIVE/NITROSATIVE STRESS PROFILE

NFκB

- CML
- ROS
- NOX nitrotyrosine
- TBARS
- 8-Keto $PGF_2\alpha$
- 8-OH, guanosine

TEST PROTOCOL

- Vitamin E
- Vitamin C
- Plasma antioxidant capacity
- Superoxide anion

Patient Preparation

Patient should fast for 10 to 12 hours prior to collection of specimen. Patient should not be on any medications that influence insulin production or secretion, if possible.

Specimen Collection

After a 12-hour fast, collect blood by venipuncture into 10-mL sampling vials containing NH_4 and 2.7-mL vials containing EDTA (final concentration 0.1%). Obtain plasma by centrifugation at 1500g at room temperature for 10 minutes. Immediately store samples of plasma from EDTA vials at -850°C for subsequent analysis (vitamins and antioxidant capacity). For F_2 isoprostane analysis, aliquots (1 jl) of plasma from vials containing NH_4 are combined with 10 µL of chain-breaking antioxidant butylated hydroxytoluene at a final concentration of 25 µmol/L and stored at –850°C until analysis.

Special Specimens

For tumor/tissue and various fluids (e.g., CSF, peritoneal fluid, synovial fluid) contact ISI for requirements and special handling instructions.

Shipping Instructions

Specimens should be shipped frozen in dry ice.

References

1. Ziegler D, Sohr C, Nourooz-Zadeh J. Oxidative stress and antioxidant defense in relation to the severity of diabetic polyneuropathy and cardiovascular autonomic neuropathy. Diabetes Care. Sep;27(9):2178-83, 2004
2. Tripathy D, Mohanty P, Dhindsa S, et al. Elevation of free fatty acids induces inflammation and impairs vascular reactivity in healthy subjects. Diabetes. Dec;52(12):2882-7, 2003.
3. Dhindsa S, Tripathy D, Mohanty P, et al. Differential effects of glucose and alcohol on reactive oxygen species generation and intranuclear nuclear factor-kappaB in mononuclear cells. Metabolism. Mar;53(3):330-4, 2004.

CPT Codes:
Lipid Peroxide (for TBARS, Thiobarbituric Acid Reactive Substances) 82491
Unspecified Immunoassay 83519

PANCREATIC FUNCTION SCREEN

BLOOD
- Trypsin
- Amylase
- Lipase
- Elastase

SERUM
- Amylase
- Lipase
- Trypsin

STOOL
- Fat
- Chymotrypsin
- Elastase-1

Patient Preparation

Patient should fast for 10 to 12 hours prior to collection of specimen. Antacid medications and medications affecting intestinal motility or pancreatic function should be discontinued, if possible, for at least 48 hours prior to collection.

Specimen Requirements

BLOOD
Collect 10 mL serum or EDTA plasma and separate as soon as possible. Freeze plasma immediately after separation. Minimum specimen size is 3 mL.

STOOL
See complete fecal collection instructions in the introduction to Chapter 3.

CPT Codes: Serum
Amylase 82150
Lipase 83690
Trypsin 84488
Elastase 83519
Pancreatic Elastase-1 82656
CPT Codes: Basal
Fecal Fat • Quantitative 82710 • Qualitative 82705
Fecal Elastase-1 82656
Fecal Chymotrypsin 84311

Shipping Instructions

Specimens should be shipped frozen in dry ice.

References

1. Hahn JU, Bochnig S, Kerner W, et al. A new fecal elastase 1 test using polyclonal antibodies for the detection of exocrine pancreatic insufficiency. Pancreas. Mar;30(2):189-91, 2005.
2. Luth S, Teyssen S, Forssmann K, et al. Fecal elastase-1 determination: 'gold standard' of indirect pancreatic function tests? Scand J Gastroenterol. Oct;36(10):1092-9, 2001.
3. Gullo L, Ventrucci M, Tomassetti P, et al. Fecal elastase 1 determination in chronic pancreatitis. Dig Dis Sci. Jan;44(1):210-3, 1999.

POLYCYSTIC OVARY SYNDROME (PCOS) SCREEN

The following measurements are required for the diagnosis of polycystic ovary disease:

BLOOD

- Total and free testosterone
- SHBG
- Dehydroepiandrosterone sulfate (DHEA-S)
- Prolactin
- LH/FSH (frequent but not required)
- TSH
- 17α-Hydroxy progesterone
- Glucose (fasting)
- Insulin
- C-peptide

Patient Preparation

Patient should fast for 10 to 12 hours prior to collection of specimen. Patient should not be on any medications that influence insulin production or secretion or any corticosteroid, ACTH, thyroid, estrogen, or gonadotropin medications, if possible, for at least 48 hours prior to collection.

Specimen Requirements

Collect 10 mL serum or EDTA plasma and separate as soon as possible. Freeze serum or plasma immediately after separation. Minimum specimen size is 4 mL.

Shipping Instructions

Specimens should be shipped frozen in dry ice.

References

1. Zawadzski JK, Dunaif A. Diagnostic criteria for polycystic ovary syndrome: towards a rational approach. In: Dunaif A, Givens J, Haseltine F, Merriam G, eds. Polycystic Ovary Syndrome. Boston: Blackwell Scientific; 1992:377-84.

CPT Codes:
Total and Free Testosterone 84403, 84402
Sex Hormone–Binding Globulin 84270
Dehydroepiandrosterone Sulfate (DHEA-S) 82627
Prolactin 84146
LH/FSH (Frequent but Not Required) 83002/83001
TSH 84443
17α-Hydroxy Progesterone 83498
Glucose (Fasting) 82947
Insulin 83525
C-Peptide 84681
PCOS 82627, 83001, 83002, 84402, 84403

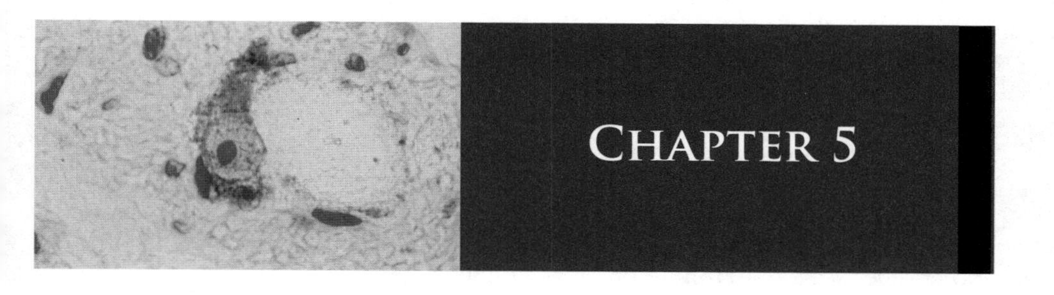

DYNAMIC CHALLENGE PROTOCOLS, INCLUDING CPT CODES

RATIONALE FOR DYNAMIC CHALLENGE PROTOCOLS

Careful evaluation of GI and pancreatic disorders involves a multiplicity of interrelated factors governed by a number of hormonal axes with varying degrees of interdependence. From this composite view of interdependency, these challenge protocols are designed to help elucidate specific GI, pancreatic, and neuroendocrine abnormalities. Emphasis is placed on stimulation and/or suppression tests designed to exploit the failure of normal homeostatic regulation through metabolic pathways.

These challenge protocols represent guidelines in evaluating a variety of GI-related syndromes. The listings are selected to provide maximal information, usefulness, and significance for interpretation in the endocrine workup of the patient or research subject.

Important Notes

No patient should undergo a dynamic challenge protocol without the direct and constant supervision of trained medical personnel. The doses listed for the following protocols are intended as guidelines only. The actual dose and collection schedule must be approved by the patient's physician.

CALCIUM STIMULATION FOR GASTRINOMA

Test, Times of Collection

Gastrin: fasting; 1, 2, and 3 hours

Stimulus/Challenge

Following an overnight fast (after 10:00 PM), the patient should be given 15 mg elemental calcium per kilogram body weight in 500 mL saline. This should be infused over a 4-hour period with continuous cardiac monitoring.

Important Precautions

If secretin is available, avoid performing the calcium infusion test. The calcium infusion test is potentially dangerous and can induce cardiac arrhythmias and standstill if infused too quickly.

Patients undergoing dynamic challenge should be under the direct and constant supervision of medical staff at all times. Continuous cardiac monitoring is mandatory.

Specimen Requirements

In adults, collect 10 mL whole blood in a green-topped EDTA tube. Separate plasma and freeze immediately. Carefully label tubes with time of collection and patient data.

Shipping Instructions

Specimens should be shipped frozen in dry ice.

Expected Response

Gastrin response should increase by more than 100 pg/mL or by more than 50% over baseline when this level is abnormal.

References

1. DuFour DR, Gaskin JH, Jubiz WA. Dynamic procedures in endocrinology. In: Becker KL, ed. Principles and Practice of Endocrinology and Metabolism. Philadelphia: JB Lippincott Company; 1990:1762-75.
2. Alsever RN, Gotlin RW. Handbook of Endocrine Tests in Adults and Children. Chicago: Year Book Medical Publishers, Inc.; 1978.
3. Trudeau WI, McGuigan JE. Effects of calcium on serum gastrin levels in the Zollinger-Ellison syndrome. N Engl J Med. 16 Oct;281(16):862-6, 1969.

CPT Codes:
Gastrin 82941
Calcium-Pentagastrin Stimulation 80410

INSULIN HYPOGLYCEMIA PROVOCATION OF PANCREATIC POLYPEPTIDE AS A TEST FOR VAGAL INTEGRITY

Test, Times of Collection

Pancreatic polypeptide: fasting; 15, 30, 45, 60, 90, and 120 minutes after injection of insulin

Stimulus/Challenge

Following an overnight absolute fast, patient should be given 0.2 U insulin per kilogram body weight.

Important Precautions

Patients undergoing dynamic challenge should be under the direct and constant supervision of medical staff at all times. The dosages listed are intended as a guideline only. The actual dosage and collection schedule must be approved by the patient's physician.

Specimen Requirements

Collect 3 mL serum or EDTA plasma at indicated times and separate as soon as possible. Freeze specimens immediately after separation. Minimum specimen size is 1 mL per specimen collected. Specimens should be clearly identified by time of collection.

Shipping Instructions

Specimens should be shipped frozen in dry ice.

Expected Response

Pancreatic polypeptide response should increase at least 2 times over baseline level.

Interpretation

Patients with impaired pancreatic function show little or no increase in pancreatic polypeptide levels. Patients with pancreatitis or diabetes mellitus often have exaggerated responses.

Contraindications, Interferences, Drug Effects

Patients with seizure disorders on dexamethasone or more than 30 mg/day of hydrocortisone or an equivalent other short-acting glucocorticoid (7.5 mg/day prednisone or 6 mg/day methylprednisolone) may have subnormal responses without any permanent hypothalamic-pituitary-adrenal disorder.

Patients with elevated baseline levels of pancreatic polypeptide (seen in some cases of Verner-Morrison syndrome) often have decreased responses.

CPT Code:
Pancreatic Polypeptide 83519

References

1. DuFour DR, Gaskin JH, Jubiz WA. Dynamic procedures in endocrinology. In: Becker KL, ed. Principles and Practice of Endocrinology and Metabolism. Philadelphia: JB Lippincott Company; 1990:1762-75.
2. Levitt NS, Vinik AI, Sive AA, et al. Impaired pancreatic polypeptide responses to insulin-induced hypoglycemia in diabetic autonomic neuropathy. J Clin Endocrinol Metab. 50(3):445-9, 1980.

Insulin Hypoglycemia Provocation of Growth Hormone, ACTH and Cortisol (Insulin Tolerance Test)

Test, Times of Collection

Glucose, growth hormone, and/or ACTH and/or cortisol: fasting; 15, 30, 45, 60, 90, and 120 minutes

Stimulus/Challenge

Following an overnight fast (calorie-free liquids allowed) with the last dose of prednisone or hydrocortisone at 6:00 PM the prior evening or of dexamethasone 24 or more hours earlier, administer 0.1 to 0.15 U per kilogram body weight, depending on suspicion of adrenal insufficiency (use 0.1 U/kg) and adiposity (BMI >30 use 0.15 U/kg) intravenous push of regular, lispro, aspart, or glulysine insulin. Fingerstick blood glucose levels can be used to assist in determining adequacy of hypoglycemia (blood glucose <45 mg/dL or <50 mg/dL if the patient is symptomatic [e.g., diaphoretic, tremulous, light headed, anxious; experiencing facial paresthesias, altered vision]. An additional dose of insulin should be given after 30 minutes if the target glucose level is not achieved. If the nadir glucose level occurs after 30 minutes, additional blood samples are indicated to encompass the added time. Glucose, both for oral consumption and as dextrose 50%, should be available and can be given immediately upon achieving a satisfactory endpoint (i.e., hypoglycemic symptoms or hypoglycemia). Intravenous dextrose should be reserved for the rare patient who is not able to safely swallow.

Important Precautions

Patients undergoing dynamic challenge should be under the direct and constant supervision of medical staff at all times. The dosages listed are intended as a guideline only. The actual dosage and collection schedule must be approved by the patient's physician.

Specimen Requirements

Collect 10 mL serum and 10 mL EDTA plasma at indicated times and separate as soon as possible. Freeze specimens immediately after separation. Minimum specimen size is 1 mL per specimen collected. Specimens should be clearly identified by time of collection.

Shipping Instructions

Specimens should be shipped frozen in dry ice.

Expected Response

Normal GH response: increase to 4 ng/mL or higher
Normal cortisol response: increase to 18 µg/mL or higher
Normal ACTH response: >35 pg/mL

Interpretation

Patients with impaired pituitary or adrenal function fail to achieve cortisol levels above 18 μg/mL, whereas primary adrenal failure patients have elevated baseline ACTH levels. Patients with both GH and ACTH/cortisol inadequacy probably will be panhypopituitary with additional TSH/free thyroxine and gonadotropin/sex steroid inadequacy.

Contraindications, Interferences, Drug Effects

Patients with seizure disorders on dexamethasone or more than 30 mg/day hydrocortisone or equivalent other short-acting glucocorticoid (7.5 mg/day prednisone or 6 mg/day methylprednisolone) may have subnormal responses without any permanent hypothalamic-pituitary-adrenal disorder.

Reference

1. Please refer to www.endotext.com/neuroendo/neuroendo7/neuroendoframe7.htm.

CPT Codes:
ACTH 82024
Cortisol 82533
Glucose Tolerance Test 82951
Glucose Tolerance Test (each additional beyond three specimens) 82952
Growth Hormone 83003

Meal (Sham Feeding) Stimulation for Vagal Integrity

Test, Times of Collection

Pancreatic polypeptide: fasting; 30, 45, 60, 90, and 120 minutes after meal

Stimulus/Challenge

Following an overnight absolute fast, give patient 100 g of roast beef or other protein-rich meal or undergo sham feeding (i.e., chew food and spit out without swallowing).

Important Precautions

Patients undergoing dynamic challenge should be under the direct and constant supervision of medical staff at all times. The dosages listed are intended as a guideline only. The actual dosage and collection schedule must be approved by the patient's physician.

Specimen Requirements

Collect 3 mL serum or EDTA plasma at indicated times and separate as soon as possible. Freeze specimens immediately after separation. Minimum specimen size is 1 mL per specimen collected. Specimens should be clearly identified by time of collection.

Shipping Instructions

Specimens should be shipped frozen in dry ice.

Expected Response

Pancreatic polypeptide response should increase 2 to 5 times over baseline level.

Interpretation

Patients with impaired pancreatic function show little or no increase in pancreatic polypeptide levels. Patients with pancreatitis or diabetes mellitus often have exaggerated responses. Patients with duodenal ulcers frequently have elevated baseline levels of pancreatic polypeptide and exhibit a reduced response.

Contraindications, Interferences, Drug Effects

Patients with elevated baseline levels of pancreatic polypeptide (seen in some cases of Verner-Morrison syndrome) often have decreased responses.

References

1. DuFour DR, Gaskin JH, Jubiz WA. Dynamic procedures in endocrinology. In: Becker KL, ed. Principles and Practice of Endocrinology and Metabolism. Philadelphia, PA: JB Lippincott Company; 1990:1762-75.
2. Glaser B, Vinik AI, Sive AA, et al. Evidence for extravagal cholinergic mechanisms regulating pancreatic endocrine function. Diabetes. 28:434, 1979.

CPT Code:
Pancreatic Polypeptide 83519

Octreotide Suppression Test for Carcinoid and Islet Cell Tumors

Octreotide acetate and a variety of other somatostatin type 2–receptor binding analogs such as lanreotide and vapreotide have been effectively used to control symptoms, improve biochemical abnormalities caused by excessive peptide/amine release from NETs, and arrest tumor growth. Octreotide acetate is currently the only commercially available somatostatin analog approved in the United States for the treatment of NETs. Octreotide acetate is available in aqueous and sustained-release formulations (LAR).

Biochemical response:

- The aqueous form of octreotide achieves peak blood levels within 60 to 120 minutes after injection.
- Injection of the sustained-release product achieves peak blood levels in 2 weeks and may require up to three injections at monthly intervals to achieve steady-state blood levels.

Symptom responsiveness can often be predicted by an OctreoScan® in which octreotide is taken up by tumors expressing somatostatin type 2 receptors or by obtaining tissue showing the presence of somatostatin type 2 receptors in the tumor.

A surrogate measure of the potential durability of the response of the clinical syndrome to octreotide therapy is the suppression of the target hormone by octreotide in the acute test.

Patient Preparation

Acute Suppression Test

In islet cell tumor patients, following an overnight absolute fast 10 to 12 hours prior to the test, determine a baseline level by measuring the dominant peptide: in gastrinoma patients measure gastrin; in glucagonoma patients measure glucagon; in VIPoma patients measure VIP; in patients with a nonfunctional tumor measure pancreatic polypeptide levels; in aldosterone-producing adrenal tumor patients measure aldosterone. Patients should fast 1 hour prior to the test (administered in a supine position) to measure aldosterone levels.

Following the determination of the fasting baseline value, an injection of octreotide or other somatostatin analog is given in the physician's office. In the United States, 100 µg of octreotide acetate is given subcutaneously and the marker value re-measured at 1 and 2 hours after the injection.

Interpretation

A decrease of 50% in the marker value at 1 to 2 hours predicts a durable response in symptoms to long-term therapy with octreotide.

Chronic Suppression Test (of Production of Serotonin and Its Metabolites)

In carcinoid patients, following a nonfasting but diet-controlled regimen, determine a baseline level marker by measuring CGA and 24-hour urinary 5-HIAA as the biomarkers.

Subsequent to determining the 24-hour urine measurement, initiate a 3-day course of octreotide (100 µg subcutaneously three times daily). The 24-hour urinary collection is repeated on the third day. A decrease of 50% in the baseline marker value predicts a good biochemical response to long-term therapy with octreotide acetate or other somatostatin type 2–preferring analogs.

Specimen Requirements

BLOOD

Collect 10 mL EDTA plasma in a special tube containing the GI Preservative and separate as soon as possible. Freeze plasma immediately after separation. Minimum specimen size is 2 mL. Special GI Preservative tubes are available from ISI for the VIP and glucagon assays. Three-milliliter serum or EDTA plasma specimens obtained at 60 and 120 minutes following the injection may be submitted for other assays not requiring the GI Preservative.

URINE

Patients should not partake of the following foods for 48 hours prior to collection of urine for measurement of 5-HIAA and 5-HTP:

- Red wine
- Cheese
- Hot dogs
- Chocolates
- Vanilla-containing foods (e.g., ice cream)
- Custard
- Pineapple, kiwi, bananas, cassava

Shipping Instructions

Specimens should be shipped frozen in dry ice.

CPT Codes: Blood
Aldosterone 82088
Gastrin 82941, 82938
Glucagon 82943
VIP 84586
Chromogranin A 86316

CPT Codes: Urine
5-HIAA Random Urine 83497, 82570
5-HIAA 24-Hour Urine 83497

References

1. Mozell EJ, Woltering EA, O'Dorisio TM, et al. Effect of somatostatin analog on peptide release and tumor growth in the Zollinger-Ellison syndrome. Surg Gynecol Obstet. Jun;170(6):476-84, 1990.
2. Mozell EJ, Woltering EA, O'Dorisio TM, et al. Adult onset nesidioblastosis: response of glucose, insulin, and secondary peptides to therapy with Sandostatin. Am J Gastroenterol. Feb;85(2):181-8, 1990.
3. Mozell EJ, Cramer AJ, O'Dorisio TM, et al. Long-term efficacy of octreotide in the treatment of Zollinger-Ellison syndrome. Arch Surg. Sep;127(9):1019-24, discussion 1024-6, 1992.

ORAL GLUCOSE TOLERANCE TEST FOR DIABETES, INSULINOMA, IMPAIRED GLUCOSE TOLERANCE, METABOLIC SYNDROME, PCOS, REACTIVE HYPOGLYCEMIA, AND ACROMEGALY

Test, Times of Collection

Diabetes: measure glucose and insulin at 0, 30, 60, 90, and 120 minutes
Reactive hypoglycemia: measure glucose and insulin at 0, 30, 60, 90, 120, 180, 240, and 300 minutes.

Acromegaly: measure growth hormone and glucose at 0, 30, 60, 90, 120, 180, 240, and 300 minutes

Stimulus/Challenge

Glucose: 75 g orally
Pregnant patients: 100 g orally.

Expected Responses

Normal fasting glucose: <100 mg/dL
Normal peak glucose: <200 mg/dL
Normal 2h glucose: <140 mg/dL
Impaired fasting glucose: ≥100 mg/dL
Impaired glucose tolerance (IGT or prediabetes): fasting glucose >100 mg/dL, peak >200 mg/dL and 2 hours postchallenge 141–198 mg/dL)
Diabetes: fasting glucose >125 mg/dL on 2 occasions or 2-hour glucose >200 mg/dL after oral glucose in nonpregnant patients
Reactive hypoglycemia: <40 mg/dL between 2 and 5 hours postchallenge
Normal growth hormone: <1.4 ng/mL after oral glucose
Reactive hypoglycemia: <40 mg/dL between 2 and 5 hours postchallenge

Expected Response

- Fasting insulin: 5–19 µU/mL
- Insulin should increase to at least double the baseline level and at least 10 µU/mL above baseline level
- Peak levels at 30 minutes: 50–150 µU/mL
- Return to fasting at 2 hours

A lack of a rise in serum insulin after glucose is indicative of pancreatic beta cell dysfunction. Glucose levels should be monitored to ensure validation of glucose loading. Glucose levels between 140 and 200 mg/dL indicate impaired pancreatic function. Glucose levels greater than 200 mg/dL may be indicative of diabetes. A fasting insulin/glucose ratio greater than 0.25 is presumptive for insulinoma. Proinsulin/insulin ratio greater than 0.30 is also indicative of insulinoma. Growth hormone suppresses to less than 2 ng/mL in healthy people and in patients with well-controlled acromegaly.

Insulin Resistance and Beta Cell Function

Beta cell function and insulin resistance is assessed by the HOMA model developed by Mathews using the following equations:

HOMA IR = Fasting Insulin (µU/mL) x Fasting Glucose (mmol/L)/22.5
HOMA B = Fasting Insulin (µU/mL)/[Fasting Glucose (mmol/L) – 3.5]

Insulin secretory index is assessed by the following equation:

Inuslin secretory index = [Insulin 30 min (pmol/L) – Insulin 0 min (pmol/L)]/
[Glucose 30 min (mmol/L) – Glucose 0 min (mmol/L)]

Insulin secretory index/HOMA IR ratio is used to assess insulin efficacy index. Growth hormone levels should become undetectable within 1 to 2 hours of glucose challenge.

Important Precautions

Patients undergoing dynamic challenge should be under the direct and constant supervision of medical staff at all times. The dosages listed are intended as a guideline only. The actual dosage and collection schedule must be approved by the patient's physician.

Specimen Requirements

Collect 3 mL serum or EDTA plasma at indicated times and separate as soon as possible. Freeze specimens immediately after separation. Minimum specimen size is 1 mL per specimen collected. Specimens should be clearly identified by time of collection.

Shipping Instructions

Specimens should be shipped frozen in dry ice.

Contraindications, Interferences, Drug Effects

Glucose levels are higher in the evening hours than in the morning hours. Glucose levels also increase with age and obesity. Pregnancy, low-carbohydrate diet, stress, contraceptives, glucocorticoids, clofibrate, thiazides, diphenylhydantoin, caffeine, ranitidine, and propanolol may increase response. Smoking, guanethidine, and salicylates may decrease response. The test should be discontinued if patient experiences vasovagal symptoms. The test should not be given to patients with glucose intolerance (i.e., those with elevated baseline glucose levels). There is also some risk of hyperosmolality.

References

1. Fajans SS, Vinik AI. Diagnosis and treatment of "insulinoma." In: Santen RJ, Manni A, eds. Diagnosis and Management of Endocrine-Related Tumors. Boston, MA: Martinus Nijhoff Publishers; 1984:235.
2. Vinik AI, Perry RR. Neoplasms of the gastroenteropancreatic endocrine system. In: Holland JF, Bast RC Jr, Morton DL, et al, eds. Cancer Medicine, vol. 1. 4th ed. Baltimore: Williams & Wilkins; 1997:1605-41.
3. American Diabetes Association. Standards of Medical Care in Diabetes. Diabetes Care. 28:S4-S36, 2005.
4. Meyer CJ, Bogardus C, Mott DM, et al. The natural history of insulin secretory dysfunction and insulin resistance in the pathogenesis of type 2 diabetes mellitus. J Clin Invest. 104:787-97, 1999.
5. UK Prospective Diabetes Study Group, U.K. prospective diabetes study 16: overview of 6 years' therapy of type II diabetes: a progressive disease. Diabetes. Nov;44(11):1249-58, 1995.
6. Buchanan TA, Xiang AH, Peters RK, et al. Preservation of pancreatic beta-cell function and prevention of type 2 diabetes by

pharmacological treatment of insulin resistance in high-risk Hispanic women. Diabetes. 51:2796–803, 2002.
7. Porter LE, Freed MI, Jone NP, et al. Rosiglitazone improves beta-cell function as measured by proinsulin/insulin ratio in patients with type 2 diabetes [abstract]. Diabetes. 49(Suppl 1):A122, 2000.
8. Mathews DR, Hosker JP, Rudenski AS, et al. Homeostasis model assessment: insulin resistance and beta-cell function from fasting plasma glucose and insulin concentrations in man. Diabetologia. 28:412-9, 1985.
9. DuFour DR, Gaskin JH, Jubiz WA. Dynamic procedures in endocrinology. In: Becker KL, ed. Principles and Practice of Endocrinology and Metabolism. Philadelphia: JB Lippincott Company; 1990:1762-75.
10. Alsever RN, Gotlin RW. Handbook of Endocrine Tests in Adults and Children. Chicago: Year Book Medical Publishers, Inc.; 1978.
11. Rosenbloom AL, Wheeler L, Bianchi R. Age-adjusted analysis of insulin responses during normal and abnormal glucose tolerance tests in children and adolescents. Diabetes. Sep;24(9):820-8, 1975.

CPT Codes:
Glucose Tolerance Test 82951
Glucose Tolerance Test (each additional beyond three specimens) 82952
Growth Hormone 83003
Insulin-like Growth Factor Binding Protein-3 83519
Insulin-like Growth Factor-1 84305
Insulin 80422, 80432–80435 • Antibody 86337 • Blood 83525 • Free 83527

PENTAGASTRIN STIMULATION TEST FOR CALCITONIN (MEDULLARY CARCINOMA OF THE THYROID)

The pentagastrin stimulation test is used to identify patients with MCT who have normal baseline levels of calcitonin. It is also useful to identify members of a family with a known familial form of MEN-II and MCT. Pentagastrin normally stimulates the secretion of calcitonin from the C cell. Women may not respond due to the presence of estrogens. The response in persons with MCT is an exaggeration of the normal response to pentagastrin.

Stimulus/Challenge

Pentagastrin: 0.5 µg/kg body weight by intravenous bolus injection.

Times of Collection

Calcitonin: 0, 1, 2, 5, and 10 minutes

Important Precautions

Patients undergoing dynamic challenge should be under the direct and constant supervision of medical staff at all times.

Specimen Collection

Collect 3 mL serum or EDTA plasma and separate as soon as possible. Freeze specimen immediately after separation. Minimum specimen size is 1 mL.

Expected Response in Patients With Medullary Carcinoma of the Thyroid

Normal basal or fasting calcitonin levels are less than 50 pg/mL. Healthy people do not experience an increase in calcitonin above 200 pg/mL with the administration of pentagastrin.

Interpretation

An exaggerated response is seen in patients with MCT and in C cell hyperplasia. Patients with elevated basal or pentagastrin-stimulated calcitonin levels should receive screening for the RET protooncogene. Carcinoembryonic antigen measurements may be helpful in determining tumor mass.

Contraindications, Interferences, Drug Effects

Patients should be warned that they will experience transient (<1–2 minutes) flushing, nausea, chest pain, and sweating with feelings of impending doom after the administration of pentagastrin, but these resolve within minutes.

References

1. DuFour DR, Gaskin JH, Jubiz WA. Dynamic procedures in endocrinology. In: Becker KL, ed. Principles and Practice of Endocrinology and Metabolism. Philadelphia: JB Lippincott Company; 1990:1762-75.
2. Alsever RN, Gotlin RW. Handbook of Endocrine Tests in Adults and Children. Chicago: Year Book Medical Publishers, Inc.; 1978.
3. Wells SA Jr, Baylin SB, Linehan WM, et al. Provocative agents and the diagnosis of medullary carcinoma of the thyroid gland. Ann Surg. Aug;188(2):139-41, 1978.

CPT Codes:
Calcium-Pentagastrin Stimulation 80410
Calcitonin 82308

PITUITARY AND HYPOTHALAMIC DISORDERS TESTS

First-Line Screening

1. Urinary free cortisol (three 24-hour collections if suspicion exists and one or more collections are normal due to "cyclic Cushing's disease." In preclinical Cushing's syndrome, urinary free cortisol may be normal.
2. Low-dose dexamethasone suppression test, either overnight (1 mg between 11:00 PM and 12:00 AM) or 0.5 mg every 6 hours for 48 hours. N1 suppression is to less than 1.8 µg/dL (50 nmol/L).
3. Circadian rhythm of cortisol: obtain serum cortisols at 8:00 AM to 09:30 AM, 4:30 PM to 6:00 PM, and 11:00 PM to 12:00 AM. The latter samples can be obtained with the patient asleep as an inpatient after 48 hours, but only if not acutely ill. Alternatively, the patient can test at home with collections of salivary cortisol.

Second-Line Testing

1. Circadian rhythm of cortisol: see above.
2. Low-dose dexamethasone suppression: 0.5 mg every 6 hours for 48 hours with measurement of 24-hour urine free cortisol on the second day. Excretion of <10 µg/24 hours (27 nmol/L) is normal.
3. Dexamethasone suppression test with CRH stimulation: low-dose DST (0.5 mg every 6 hours for 48 hours followed by 100 µg or 1 µg/kg of ovine CRH intravenously. Cortisol response >1.4 µg/dL at 15 minutes is consistent with Cushing's disease.

References

1. Arnaldi G, Angeli A, Atkinson AB, et al. Diagnosis and complications of Cushing's syndrome: a consensus statement. J Clin Endocrinol Metab. 88:5593–602, 2003
2. Raff H, Raff JI, Findling JW. Late-night salivary cortisol as a screening test for Cushing's syndrome. J Clin Endocrinol Metab. 83:2681-6, 1998.
3. Aron DC, Raff H, Findling JW. Effectiveness versus efficacy: the limited value in clinical practice of high dose dexamethasone suppression testing in the differential diagnosis of adrenocorticotropin-dependent Cushing's syndrome. J Clin Endocrinol Metab. 82:1780-5, 1997.

CPT Codes:
11-Deoxycortisol, Urine 82634
Cortisol, Serum 82533
Cortisol Level, Urine 83519
Dexamethasone, Serum 83516

PROVOCATIVE PANCREATIC EXOCRINE FUNCTION TESTS

The secretin-cholecystokinin stimulation test measures the concentration and output of bicarbonate, lipase, and trypsin in the duodenal juice. This test is the gold standard for determining the degree of pancreatic exocrine insufficiency, but it is seldom done in the clinical settings. Most institutions depend on the indirect assessment of pancreatic exocrine insufficiency by determining the presence and severity of fecal steatorrhea and/or by direct pancreatic enzyme measurement.

References for Acute Pancreatitis

1. Rettally CA, Skarda S, Garza MA, et al. The usefulness of laboratory tests in the early assessment of severity of acute pancreatitis. Crit Rev Clin Lab Sci. Apr;40(2):117-49, 2003.
2. Smotkin J, Tenner S. Laboratory diagnostic tests in acute pancreatitis. J Clin Gastroenterol. Apr;34(4):459-62, 2002.

References for Chronic Pancreatitis

1. Lankisch PG. The problem of diagnosing chronic pancreatitis. Dig Liver Dis. Mar;35(3):131-4, 2003.
2. Go VLW. Exocrine pancreatic secretion and insufficiency. In: Barkin JS, Lo SK, eds. The Use of Pancreatic Enzymes: Proceedings of a Faculty Symposium. Ghent, NY: Galen Press; 2003:2-6.
3. Owyang C, Vinik A. Physiology of the exocrine pancreas. In: Dent TL, ed. Pancreatic Disease, Diagnosis and Therapy. New York: Grune and Stratton; 1981:15.

CPT Code:
Gastrin After Secretin Stimulation 82938

Provocative Tests for Dumping Syndrome

Dumping occurs following surgical procedures that extirpate or inactivate the pylorus. Two forms of dumping occur: early dumping is characterized by shock-like symptoms, and late dumping is characterized by symptoms of hypoglycemia

Stimulus/Challenge

Following baseline blood draw, the patient is given a carbohydrate-rich, high-calorie breakfast consisting of two eggs, two strips of bacon, two pieces of whole wheat toast, and a serving of ice cream topped with flavored syrup. This test meal contains 750 kcal, 21 g protein, 30 g fat, and 99 g of carbohydrate. The meal should be ingested within 10 minutes to evoke the maximum response.

Timing of Blood Draws

Collect 5 mL of whole blood in green-topped EDTA tubes at 10, 15, 30, 45, 60, 120, and 180 minutes following completion of the meal. Glucose levels and the hormones listed below should be measured. In patients with late dumping, additional blood samples should be collected at after the test meal.

Hormones Assayed

Insulin, C-peptide, motilin, pancreatic polypeptide, GLP-1

Specimen Requirements

Whole blood should immediately be separated and the plasma frozen.

Shipping Instructions

Specimens should be shipped frozen in dry ice.

References

1. Richards WO, Geer R, O'Dorisio TM, et al. Octreotide acetate induces fasting small bowel motility in patients with dumping syndrome. J Surg Res. Dec;49(6):483-7, 1990.
2. Geer RJ, Richards WO, O'Dorisio TM, et al. Efficacy of octreotide acetate in treatment of severe postgastrectomy dumping syndrome. Ann Surg. Dec;212(6):678-87, 1990.
3. Watson JC, O'Dorisio TM, Woltering EA. Octreotide acetate controls the peptide hypersecretion and symptoms associated with the dumping syndrome. Asian J Surg. 20:283-8, 1998.

CPT Codes:
GLP-1 Unspecified, Immunoassay 83519
C-Peptide 84681
Pancreatic Polypeptide 83519
Insulin 83525
Motilin 83519

Secretin Stimulation Test for Gastrinoma

Test, Times of Collection

Gastrin: fasting; 2, 5, 10, 15, and 30 minutes

Stimulus/Challenge

Following an overnight fast from 10:00 PM, patient should be given secretin 2 U/kg by intravenous bolus injection.

Important Precautions

Patients undergoing dynamic challenge should be under the direct and constant supervision of medical staff at all times. The doses listed are intended as a guideline only. The actual dose and collection schedule must be approved by the patient's physician.

Specimen Requirements

In adults, collect 10 mL whole blood in a green-topped EDTA tube. Separate plasma and freeze immediately. Carefully label tubes with time of collection and patient data.

Shipping Instructions

Specimens should be shipped frozen in dry ice.

Expected Response

Gastrin response should increase no more than 50% over baseline level in healthy people. In gastrinoma, the rise increase is greater than 100 pg/mL above basal levels.

Interpretation

Patients with gastrinoma exhibit elevated baseline gastrin levels and a paradoxical rise in the gastrin response to secretin greater than 100 pg/mL above their baseline level. Healthy people have a fall or no rise in gastrin levels. Patients with hypochlorhydria or achlorhydria from PPI use, type 1 gastric carcinoid, atrophic gastritis, or pernicious anemia have elevated gastrin levels (>150 pg/mL) but exhibit no response to administration of secretin. Patients with active peptic ulcers may show a 30% to 50% increase over baseline levels. Healthy patients frequently exhibit suppression in gastrin levels following secretin administration.

References

1. DuFour DR, Gaskin JH, Jubiz WA. Dynamic procedures in endocrinology. In: Becker KL, ed. Principles and Practice of Endocrinology and Metabolism. Philadelphia: JB Lippincott Company; 1990:1762-75.
2. Alsever RN, Gotlin RW. Handbook of Endocrine Tests in Adults and Children. Chicago: Year Book Medical Publishers, Inc.; 1978.
3. Feldman M, Schiller LR, Walsh JH, et al. Positive intravenous secretin test in patients with achlorhydria-related hypergastrinemia. Gastroenterology. Jul;93(1):59-62, 1987.
4. Giusti M, Sidoti M, Augeri C, et al. Effect of short-term treatment with low dosages of the proton-pump inhibitor omeprazole on serum chromogranin A levels in man. Eur J Endocrinol. Mar;150(3):299-303, 2004.

CPT Codes:
Gastrin 82938–82941
Secretin Stimulation Test 82938

72-HOUR SUPERVISED FAST FOR THE DIAGNOSIS OF INSULINOMA

A 72-hour fast is the preferred diagnostic procedure for the diagnosis of an insulinoma.

Patient Preparation

Patient should fast for 72 hours. Water and diet soft drinks without caffeine are permitted. Patients submitted to a 72-hour fast should be under the direct and constant supervision of medical staff at all times.

Test, Times of Collection

Insulin, glucose, and C-peptide samples are drawn at 0, 12, 24, 36, 48, and 72 hours after beginning fast. If the patient becomes symptomatic (i.e., documented fingerstick hypoglycemia) at any time during the test, blood should be drawn immediately for glucose, insulin, and C-peptide levels. Administer glucose and terminate the procedure.

Specimen Requirements

Collect 10 mL of whole blood in a green-topped EDTA tube. Separate plasma and freeze immediately. Carefully label 3-mL EDTA tubes with time of collection and patient data.

Shipping Instructions

Specimens should be shipped frozen in dry ice.

Interpretation

Expected response in healthy people:

- Insulin levels should decrease to less than 4 μU/mL.
- Insulin/glucose ratio should be less than 0.3.

Expected response in insulinoma:

- A fasting insulin/glucose ratio greater than 0.3 is presumptive of insulinoma.
- An elevated C-peptide level greater than 4 ng/mL in the absence of obesity and insulin resistance suggests insulinoma.

Caveats

Ketones should be present in the urine to confirm fasting. 18-Hydroxybutyrate concentrations should also be obtained with each blood draw to support or deny suppression of insulin and release of lipolysis. Suppressed C-peptide levels (<0.5 ng/mL) during fasting suggests factitious hypoglycemia. Elevated C-peptide levels may suggest suspected sulfonylurea-induced factitious hypoglycemia.

CPT Codes:
C-Peptide 84681
Glucose 82947
Insulin 83525

References

1. Fajans SS, Vinik AI. Diagnosis and treatment of "insulinoma." In: Santen RJ, Manni A, eds. Diagnosis and Management of Endocrine-Related Tumors. Boston, MA: Martinus Nijhoff Publishers; 1984:235.
2. Vinik AI, Perry RR. Neoplasms of the gastroenteropancreatic endocrine system. In: Holland JF, Bast RC Jr, Morton DL, et al, eds. Cancer Medicine, vol. 1, 4th ed. Baltimore: Williams & Wilkins; 1997:1605-41.

WATER DEPRIVATION/DESMOPRESSIN TEST FOR DIABETES INSIPIDUS: HYPOTHALAMIC (HDI), NEPHROGENIC (NDI), AND DIPSOGENIC (DDI)

If that patient has moderate polyuria (3–7 L/day), the dehydration test may be started in the evening, with the last fluid being consumed before bed. If polyuria is severe (>7 L/day), begin the test in the morning to avoid dangerous dehydration.

Patient Preparation

Patient may have free access to fluid overnight prior to test but should be cautioned to avoid caffeine and smoking. At 7:50 AM the patient voids urine, and starting weight is accurately determined on a scale that can be used throughout the procedure.

Dehydration Phase

- At 8:00 AM, measure plasma and urine osmolality and urine volume.
- Patient should fast for the duration of the test.
- Weigh patient at 2-hour intervals or after each liter of urine is excreted.
- Measure plasma and urine osmolality and urine volume every 2 hours and after each urine voided. When two consecutive measures of urine osmolality differ by no more than 10% and the patient has lost 2% of body weight, plasma is drawn for Na^+, osmolality, and vasopressin determinations.
- Stop the test if weight loss exceeds 3% of starting weight, thirst is intolerable, or serum sodium exceeds normal at anytime during the test. Plasma vasopressin is obtained at the time the test is terminated.
- Supervise patient closely to avoid undisclosed drinking.

Desmopressin (DDAVP) Phase

Inject 2 µg DDVAP intravenously/intramuscularly.

Allow patient to eat and drink up to 1.5 to 2.0 times the volume of urine voided during water deprivation.

Measure plasma and urine osmolality and urine volume hourly to 8:00 PM.

Interpretation

HDI: urine osmolality is less than 300 mOsm/kg accompanied by plasma osmolality greater than 290 mOsm/kg after dehydration; urine osmolality should rise above 750 mOsm/kg after DDAVP.

NDI: failure to increase urine osmolality above 300 mOsm/kg after dehydration with no response to DDAVP.

DDI: appropriate urine concentration during dehydration without significant rise in plasma osmolality.

If HDI is diagnosed, the next step should be imaging of the hypothalamus/perisellar region with MRI to exclude possible tumors. HDI frequently is associated with loss of the normal posterior pituitary bright spot on T1-weighted MRI, which correlates with posterior pituitary vasopressin content.

Specimen Requirements

Collect 5 mL of whole blood in green-topped EDTA tubes and separate as soon as possible. Freeze plasma immediately after separation. Urine osmolality should be determined immediately or the specimens placed in sealed containers to avoid evaporation. Freezing is appropriate if the specimen is to be stored long term.

Shipping Instructions

Specimens should be shipped frozen in dry ice.

Reference

1. Please refer to www.endotext.org.

CPT Codes:
Sodium 84295
Electrolyte Panel 80051
Osmolality 24-Hour Urine 83935
Osmolality Random Urine 83935
Osmolality Plasma 83930
Vasopressin (Antidiuretic Hormone) 84588
Urea Nitrogen, 24-Hour Urine 84540
Urea Nitrogen Clearance 84545
Urea Nitrogen Serum 84520
Urea Nitrogen and Creatinine Profile 82570, 84540

WATER LOAD TEST FOR IMPAIRED WATER CLEARANCE

Caveat

This test is safe only in a patient who has returned to a normal or near normal osmolality. In this case, the test is used chiefly to determine whether the initial problem with hyponatremia has resolved.

Patient Preparation

Patient preparation includes omitting NSAIDs, diuretics, and all other nonessential medications for 24 hours or more in patients on chlorthalidone, spironolactone, or other drugs with long half-lives. The patient should have nothing orally and not smoke for 4 hours before or during the test. After emptying the bladder, 20 mL/kg tepid water should be consumed over 30 minutes. Urine is collected hourly or whenever voided and osmolality and volume recorded. The test is completed at 4 hours. Normal response in a non–saline-depleted subject is 85% to greater than 100% excretion of the water load within 4 hours and drop in urine osmolality to near maximally dilute (i.e., <100 mOsm/kg in healthy young to middle-aged adults without renal disease).

Specimen Requirements

No blood collection is necessary. Determine urine osmolality immediately or place the specimens in sealed containers to avoid evaporation. Freezing is appropriate if specimens are to be stored long term.

Interpretation

For a full discussion on causes of impaired water clearance, see Hyponatremia and Syndrome of Inappropriate Antidiuretic Hormone in Chapter 2.

		Hypovolemia		Euvolemia		Hypervolemia	
Extracellular Na+		↓↓		→		↑	
Total body water		↓		↑		↑↑	
Common causes	• Renal loss • Diuretics • Mineralocorticoid deficiency • Salt-losing nephritis • Cerebral salt wasting		• Extra-renal loss • Vomiting • Diarrhea • Burns	• SIADH • Hypothyroidism • Glucocorticoid deficiency • Sick cell syndrome	• Cardiac failure • Cirrhosis • Nephrotic syndrome		• Renal failure
Urinary Na+ (mmol/L)	>20		<10	>20	<10		>20
Plasma osmolarity (mOsm/kg)	>280		>280	>280	<280		
Urine osmolarity (mOsm/kg)	>280		<280	>280	<280		

Reference

1. Please refer to www.endotext.org.

CPT Codes:
Sodium 84295
Electrolyte Panel 80051
Osmolality 24-Hour Urine 83935
Osmolality Random Urine 83935

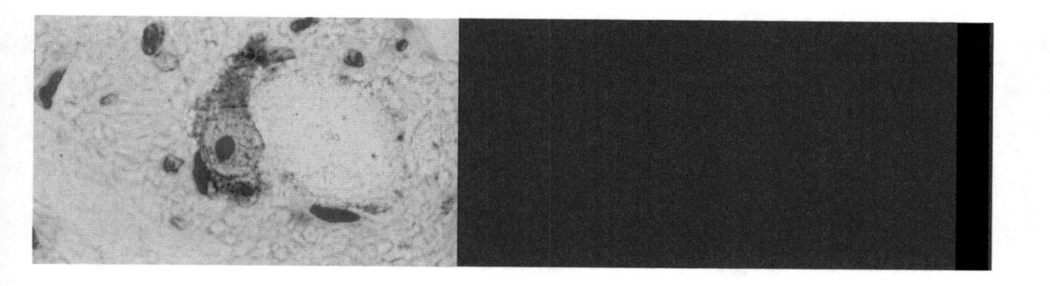

INDEX

A

D

E

F

G

H

K

L

M

N

O

P

R

S

U

V

W

Z

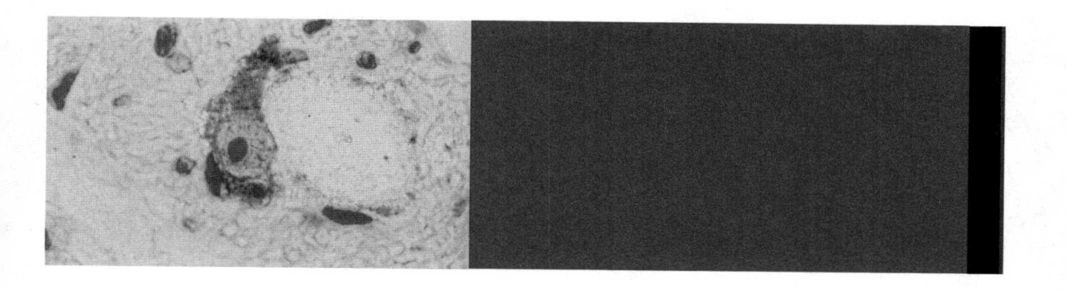

ABBREVIATIONS

ABBREVIATIONS

ACE = angiotensin-converting enzyme
ACTH = adrenocorticotropic hormone (corticotropin)
ApoE4 = apolipoprotein E4
APUD = amine precursor uptake and decarboxylation
BMI = body mass index
BNP = brain natriuretic peptide
BUN = blood urea nitrogen
CA = cancer-associated antigen
CCK = cholecystokinin
CEA = carcinoembryonic antigen
CGA = chromogranin A
CGRP = calcitonin gene–related peptide
CML = carboxy methyl lysine
CRH = corticotropin-releasing hormone
CRF = corticotropin-releasing factor
CRP = C-reactive protein
CSF = cerebrospinal fluid
CT = computed tomography
DDAVP = desmopressin acetate
DDI = dipsogenic diabetes insipidus
DHEA-S = dehydroepiandrosterone sulfate
DHK-PGE_2 = dihydroketo prostaglandin E_2
DHK-$PGF_2\alpha$ = dihydroketo prostaglandin $F_2\alpha$
DIDMOAD = diabetes insipidus, diabetes mellitus, optic atrophy, and deafness
DST = dexamethasone suppression test
DVT = deep venous thrombosis
EC = enterochromaffin
ECL = enterochromaffin-like
EDTA = ethylene amine tetraacetic acid
EIA = enzyme immunoassay
EL = elastase
ELISA = enzyme-linked immunosorbent assay
FBG = fasting blood glucose
FEV_1 = forced expiratory volume in 1 second
FFA = free fatty acid
FSH = follicle-stimulating hormone
GAD = glutamic acid decarboxylase
GEP = gastroenteropancreatic
GEP-ET = gastroenteropancreatic endocrine tumors
GERD = gastroesophageal reflux disease
GH = growth hormone (somatotropin)
GHRH = growth hormone–releasing hormone
GHS-R1a = growth hormone secretagogue type 1a
GI = gastrointestinal
GIP = gastric inhibitory polypeptide

GLP = glucagon-like peptide
GRP = gastrin-releasing peptide
α-GSU = human glycoprotein hormone alpha subunit
5-HIAA = 5-hydroxyindoleacetic acid
5-HT = 5-hydroxytryptamine (serotonin)
5-HTP = 5-hydroxytryptophan
HDI = hypothalamic (central) diabetes insipidus
HDL = high-density lipoprotein
HLA = human leukocyte antigen
HOMA IR, B = homeostasis model assessment of insulin resistance, of beta cell function
HS CRP = highly sensitive C-reactive protein
HVA = homovanillic acid
^{131}I-MIBG = iodine-131 meta-iodobenzylguanidine
IAA = insulin autoantibodies
IAPP = islet amyloid polypeptide
IBS = irritable bowel syndrome
ICA = islet cell antigen
IgA, G = immunoglobulin A, G
IGF-1, -2 = insulin-like growth factor type 1, type 2
IGT = impaired glucose tolerance
IL-1 through IL-18 = interleukin-1 through IL-18
6-Keto-PGF$_1$α = 6-keto prostaglandin F$_1$α
LAR = long-acting repeatable
LDL = low-density lipoprotein
LH = luteinizing hormone
MCT = medullary carcinoma of the thyroid
MDMA = 3,4-methylenedioxymethamphetamine
MEN-I, -II, -III = multiple endocrine neoplasia type I, type II, type III
MODY = mature-onset diabetes of youth
MRI = magnetic resonance imaging
MSH = melanocyte-stimulating hormone
NDI = nephrogenic diabetes insipidus
NET = neuroendocrine tumors
NFκB = nuclear factor kappa B
NKA = neurokinin A
NME = necrolytic migratory erythema
NMR = nuclear magnetic resonance
NPY = neuropeptide Y
NSE = neuron-specific enolase
PAI-1 = plasminogen activator inhibitor 1
PARP = polyadenosine diphosphate ribose polymerase
PCOS = polycystic ovary syndrome
PG = prostaglandin
PG-I, -II = pepsinogen I, II
PGD$_2$ = prostaglandin D$_2$
PGE$_1$ = prostaglandin E$_1$

PGE_2 = prostaglandin E_2
$PGF_1\alpha$ = prostaglandin $F_1\alpha$
$PGF_2\alpha$ = prostaglandin $F_2\alpha$
PHIM = peptide histidine isoleucine
PP = pancreatic polypeptide
PPI = proton pump inhibitors
PTH = parathyroid hormone
PTHRP = parathyroid hormone–related peptide
PYY = peptide YY
RIA = radioimmunoassay
SD = standard deviation
SHBG = sex hormone–binding globulin
SIADH = syndrome of inappropriate antidiuretic hormone secretion
SLI = somatostatin-like immunoreactivity
SRIF = somatotropin release–inhibiting factor
T3 = triiodothyronine
T4 = thyroxine
TCT = thyrocalcitonin
TNFα, β = tumor necrosis factor alpha, beta
TRH = thyrotropin-releasing hormone
TSH = thyroid-stimulating hormone
TTG = tissue transglutaminase
VIP = vasoactive intestinal polypeptide
VHL = von Hippel-Lindau
VMA = vanillyl mandelic acid
WDHHA = watery diarrhea syndrome (watery diarrhea, hypokalemia, hypochlorhydria, and acidosis)
ZE = Zollinger-Ellison syndrome

Inter Science Institute
944 West Hyde Park Blvd.
Inglewood, CA 90302

(800) 255-CURE
(800) 421-7133
(310) 677-3322

Physician, Lab, Hospital: ____________________

Address: ____________________

Department: ____________________

City: ____________________ State: ________ Zip: ________

PATIENT

Patient Name: ____________________

Age: ________ Client Acct. No.: ____________________

Sex: ________ Specimen Type: ____________________

Collection Date: ____________________

Collection Time: ________ AM ________ PM

Date Specimen Time Rec'd at ISI: ________ AM ________ PM | **ISI Accn. No.** ____________________

- ❑ AMYLIN*
- ❑ BOMBESIN*
- ❑ C-PEPTIDE
- ❑ CALCITONIN
- ❑ CHOLECYSTOKININ (CCK)*
- ❑ CHROMOGRANIN A (CgA)
- ❑ ELASTASE: ________ Serum ________ Fecal
- ❑ FREE INSULIN
- ❑ GALANIN*
- ❑ GASTRIC INHIBITORY POLYPEPTIDE (GIP)*
- ❑ GASTRIN*
- ❑ GASTRIN RELEASING PEPTIDE (GRP)*
- ❑ GHRELIN*
- ❑ GLUCAGON*
- ❑ GROWTH HORMONE RELEASING HORMONE
- ❑ HISTAMINE
- ❑ INSULIN
- ❑ INTERLEUKINS: ________
- ❑ MOTILIN*
- ❑ NEUROKININ A*
- ❑ NEUROKININ B*
- ❑ NEUROPEPTIDE K*
- ❑ NEUROPEPTIDE Y*
- ❑ NEUROTENSIN*
- ❑ OCTREOTIDE (Sandostatin®)
- ❑ PANCREASTATIN*
- ❑ PANCREATIC POLYPEPTIDE (PP)
- ❑ PEPSINOGEN I
- ❑ PEPSINOGEN II
- ❑ PEPTIDE YY*
- ❑ PHIM*
- ❑ PROSTAGLANDINS (PG): ________
- ❑ SANDOSTATIN® (Octreotide)
- ❑ SECRETIN*
- ❑ SEROTONIN (5-HT, Serum only)
- ❑ SOMATOSTATIN*
- ❑ SUBSTANCE P*
- ❑ THROMBOXANE B2
- ❑ VASOACTIVE INTESTINAL POLYPEPTIDE*

PROFILES:

- ❑ CARCINOID FOLLOW-UP SCREEN
- ❑ DIARRHEA SYNDROME
- ❑ DUMPING SYNDROME
- ❑ FLUSHING SYNDROME
- ❑ GASTRINOMA SCREEN
- ❑ POLYCYSTIC OVARY SCREEN
- ❑ PSEUDOGASTRINOMA SYNDROME

OTHER ASSAY OR PROFILE: ____________________

DYNAMIC CHALLENGE PROTOCOLS: Test(s): ____________________

Collection Time(s): ____________________

TOTAL VOLUME IS REQUIRED FOR URINE ASSAYS: ____________ / **24 hours**

* **THE FOLLOWING ASSAYS SHOULD BE COLLECTED USING THE G.I. PRESERVATIVE TUBES AVAILABLE FROM INTER SCIENCE INSTITUTE (ISI).**
(GI Preservative highly recommended to stabilize peptide integrity.)